A Practical Introduction to
CRANIAL CT

A Practical Introduction to CRANIAL CT

A. R. VALENTINE FRCR
Consultant Neuroradiologist, Royal Free Hospital, London.
Late Senior Registrar, Lysholm Radiological Dept., National
Hospital for Nervous Diseases, London

P. PULLICINO MRCP
Resident in Neurology, University of Rochester, New York.
Late Research Fellow, National Hospital for Nervous Diseases, London

E. BANNAN FRCR
Consultant Radiologist, Prince Henry Hospital, Melbourne, Australia.
Late Senior Registrar, National Hospital for Nervous Diseases, London

With a Foreword by
Professor G. H. du Boulay
Director of Lysholm Radiological Department,
National Hospital for Nervous Diseases, Queen Square, London

William Heinemann Medical Books Ltd
London

William Heinemann Medical Books Ltd.,
23 Bedford Square
London, WC1B 3HH

ISBN 0 433 33602 1

First published 1981
Reprinted 1986

Printed and bound in Great Britain at
The Camelot Press Ltd, Southampton

Contents

Acknowledgements

The authors gratefully acknowledge the help of Professor G. du Boulay, Drs B. Kendall and I. Moseley and the radiographic staff of The National Hospital for Nervous Diseases, Queen Square. We thank Dr Brian Moffatt for his help with the clinical section.

The authors are also indebted to Mrs Amanda Pink (*née* Rudden) and Mrs Wendy Cirello for expert secretarial assistance.

Foreword

Radiology is or should be concerned as much with communication as with actual diagnosis. Not only do neuroradiologists need to teach the beginner within their own discipline, there is also a universal requirement within the clinical neurosciences that CT images should be understood by all.

The radiologist, of course, controls the way in which the information is presented in the image. He also controls the acquisition of the information at the actual examination from which he subsequently selects what he believes to be relevant; but in the rush of work both written and spoken language are inadequate means of communicating the results to the clinician and of receiving back from him further amended requests for other information.

All parties need a picture or a set of measurements upon which to congregate their thoughts.

Many second generation neuroradiologists, beginning in the late 1940s and early 1950s, fled from a situation where their general radiological colleagues and teachers sat all day behind piles of films or in front of dim fluorescent screens, connected to the bedside dialogue only by a few misleading remarks on a scrap of paper. Neuroradiology offered a chance to work hand in glove with the neurologist and, more particularly, with the neurosurgeon in a proximity that led to conversation.

Service to the patient's problem came from standing around the radiographs. Now there has been a shift of practice with the universal insinuation of CT into neurology and the reintroduction of the general radiologist into significant preliminary neuroradiological work. There may even be too many examinations for individual spoken discussion to be practicable about every patient.

So almost everyone entering neurology, neurosurgery and general radiology, not just neuroradiology, needs what used to be known as a primer on the subject of CT of the central nervous system. This one has few rivals, coming as it does at a time when the rapid advances in CT technique, interpretation and diagnostic management have begun to slow down and to stabilize.

Professor George du Boulay

CHAPTER ONE

Technical Aspects

Computed tomography is the product of applying computer technology and techniques of image reconstruction to modern radiological equipment. The technology of CT is developing rapidly and where a modification to the X-ray source-detector system is sufficiently fundamental, the advance is said to give birth to a new generation of machines. However, the principles are adequately illustrated by a consideration of the early type of machine such as EMI CT 1000 (a first generation scanner).

The equipment comprises a gantry (supporting the X-ray tube and detector system), patient couch, computer system and viewing system. The fundamental processes are those of data acquisition and data processing.

DATA ACQUISITION

An X-ray source is collimated to produce a pencil beam which traverses the patient and is coupled to a radiation detector. A linear scan is taken across the patient and this results in multiple readings by the detector. The gantry then rotates (indexes) through 1° and a further linear scan takes place, repeating the multiple detector samples. This process is repeated 180 times at the end of which a huge number of detector readings are available for computer processing. This system is referred to as a translate-rotate system. Two major developments in the quest for increased data accumulation in shorter scan time have been:

1. Development of a fan beam X-ray source coupled to multiple detectors, utilizing a larger gantry index between translation (Fig. 1.1a, b) (second generation scanners).
2. Rotate – only systems using multiple detectors, coupled with the tube or in stationary banks (third and fourth generation scanners).

DATA PROCESSING

The purpose of data processing is to calculate a precise X-ray absorption

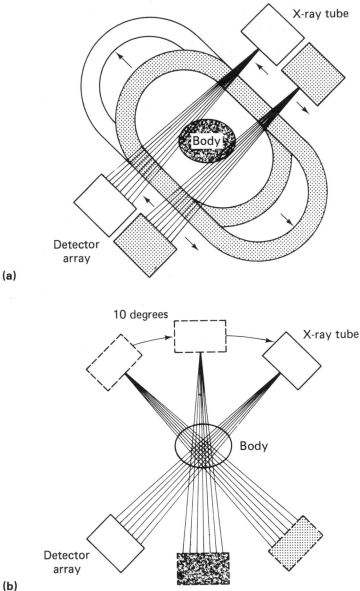

Fig. 1.1 (a)   Translate-Rotate system: movement of scanning frame during translation. (Second generation scanner.)
(b)   Translate-Rotate system: tube and detector movement during rotation. (Second generation scanner.)

(attenuation) value for each of the many individual small blocks of tissue (volume elements, voxels) which together comprise a complete tissue slice. The number of volume elements per slice is arbitrary and varies from one machine type to another, and is referred to as the matrix (Fig. 1.2). As the reconstructed image is a two-dimensional display each volume element is represented by a picture element (or pixel). The tissue area represented by each pixel is dictated by the matrix

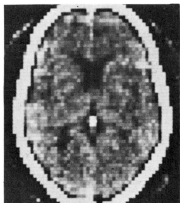

The individual picture elements are discernible in this 80 × 80 matrix image

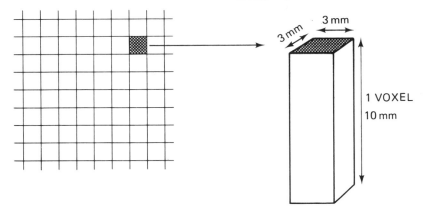

Fig. 1.2 The relationship between pixel and voxel. The image (of which only part is represented here) is made up of many picture elements (pixels). One pixel (shaded) represents a block of tissue within the scan subject. The precise dimensions of the voxel are determined by the scanner, and here relate to the CT 1000 described in the text. The 'matrix' of a machine type is a reference to the number of pixels (and therefore represented voxels) comprising the image, and is expressed as 80 × 80, 160 × 160, 320 × 320, etc. Contrast resolution increases with smaller pixel size.

The first machines resolved the data from a scan field diameter of 240 cm and slice thickness of 13 mm into an 80 × 80 matrix, such that each picture element (pixel) represented a volume element of tissue of 3 mm × 3 mm × 13 mm. Recent scanners frequently resolve the data into 160 × 160 or 320 × 320 matrix, which results in much smaller volume elements, and an increase in the number of attenuation values calculated per unit volume. Figures 1.3 and 1.4 show reconstructed images of an early 80 × 80 and recent 160 × 160 matrix. Comparison illustrates the improvement modern technology has brought to scan appearances.

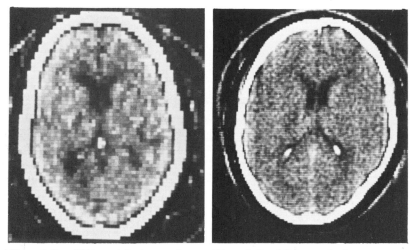

Fig. 1.3 Mid-ventricular cut. 80 × 80 matrix.

Fig. 1.4 Mid-ventricular cut. 160 × 160 matrix.

A computed numerical attenuation value is calculated for each voxel related to an arbitrary scale in which water attenuation is allocated the value 0. Two scales are in common use, employing Hounsfield units and EMI units (1 EMI unit = 2 Hounsfield units). There are 2000 units in the Hounsfield scale ranging from + 1000 to − 1000 units, and within this range are found the values of virtually all tissues encountered in diagnostic work (Table 1.1).

WINDOW LEVEL AND WIDTH

Application of a grey-scale system (of nine shades of grey between black and white) to the numerical value calculated for the constituent voxels of each slice permits a visual display of the reconstructed image. By con-

Table 1.1

Attenuation Values of Different Tissues
(Hounsfield units)

		Range	
Bone/Calcium	+ 80	–	+ 1000
Clotted blood	+ 40	–	+ 95
Grey matter	+ 36	–	+ 46
White matter	+ 22	–	+ 32
CSF	0	–	+ 8
Water		0	
Fat	– 20	–	– 100
Air		–1000	

trolling the window level on the viewing console, the grey scale can be centred on the approximate attenuation value of the tissue of interest and then by controlling the window width different ranges of other tissue attenuations can be included in the grey scale. Both level and width are under the control of the viewer. The window width straddles the window level evenly, so that at a window width of 20, pixels of values of ten units above and ten units below the window level are included in the grey scale. Pixels whose attenuation values are more than 10 units above the window level are represented by white pixels, and similarly those pixels more than 10 units below the window level are represented by black pixels. As the window width increases each shade of the grey scale encompasses a larger number of units, and a wider range of attenuation values can be viewed simultaneously. As the window width is widened and the range increases, fine discrimination between attenuation values close to each other is of course lost.

When, on the other hand, the window width is set at 1, then the grey scale is compressed to only black and white pixels. When a pixel changes from black to white therefore, the window level reading at which this change occurs represents the actual attenuation value. When measuring tissue attenuation values, inhomogeneity of the tissue may cause problems, but the mean or mode is the best measurement to take and will be approximately that at which the bulk of pixels change (rather than the first or last few).

PARTIAL VOLUME PHENOMENON

Most machines use a slice thickness of 10 or 13 mm for a standard cranial examination, so that the full examination necessitates 8 or 10 adjacent slices. Because the slices are relatively thick, each pixel in the reconstructed image represents the mean attenuation value of the constituent tissues in the voxel, which may include bone, cerebrospinal fluid and brain tissue, as well as any pathological tissues. Even a small contribution to the slice by tissue of extreme attenuation value (e.g. bone or air) may have a marked influence on the resultant attenuation value of the pixel. Thus, for example, a slice taken predominantly through cerebral substance but including a CSF space may result in the appearance of reduced attenuation of the cerebral substance. The contribution to an apparent abnormality by the partial volume phenomenon should always be considered, especially in slices which may contain tissues of significantly different attenuation.

RADIATION DOSAGE AND RESOLUTION

The quality of the reconstructed image is considered in terms of spatial and contrast resolution. Spatial resolving power is effectively limited by pixel size. Contrast resolution depends on the signal to noise ratio within the data accumulated during the scan. Spatial and contrast resolution, slice thickness and radiation dosage are interrelated thus:

$$\text{Radiation dose} \quad \propto \frac{SR^3 \times CR^2}{\text{Slice thickness}}$$

where SR = spatial resolution
CR = contrast resolution

Radiation Protection

Protection of the lens is the most important aspect of patient protection in cranial CT. If the eyes are being irradiated, as for example in orbital scanning, then the patient should be positioned prone or supine, depending on the scanner type so that the lens is furthest from the X-ray source. This simple manoeuvre reduces lens dose by a factor of approximately eight, but this method of protection only applies to translate-rotate systems.

CHAPTER TWO

Practical Aspects

If it can be assumed that:

1. Technical excellence of radiographic staff,
2. Machine reliability and efficiency, and
3. Degree of patient co-operation are assured

then two factors assume major significance in determining how usefully and efficiently a CT department functions:

(a) Patient selection
(b) Supervision of scanning

It may be seen therefore, that in conventional departments one major factor depends mainly on the clinician while the other involves the radiologist. The logical conclusion is that intelligent co-operation leads to best patient care.

PATIENT SELECTION AND HANDLING

Patient selection is an area in which misunderstanding occurs between referring clinician and CT staff, and this may usually be avoided by better communication. The clinician may refer a patient to scan with a diagnosis of dementia. The CT scan department has great difficulty in dealing with a confused patient who is totally unable to co-operate, and the poor quality of the resulting scan reflects the lack of communication.

Dealing with patients who are unable to co-operate is a frequent experience in the CT department. The clinician should anticipate problems and recognise those patients in whom sedation or anaesthesia may be necessary and initiate such procedures prior to scanning so that delay in the department may be minimised.

The risk involved in such measures must be assessed in the clinical context and the radiologist can contribute useful advice. If exclusion of hydrocephalus, or demonstration of gross haemorrhage is sufficient information then gentle patient restraint may suffice. A fast scan option is available on many machines and this may give sufficient information to avoid general anaesthesia or hazardous sedation, even though the image is degraded. In such situations clinico-radiological collaboration can only be in the patient's best interests.

RADIOLOGICAL SUPERVISION

Supervision of CT scanning should be a 'dynamic' process and this implies a willingness to interrupt a so-called 'routine' scan at any stage to elucidate any doubtful point. In the ideal situation, the radiologist will be aware of the implications of the symptoms and signs in structural terms, and be aware of the differential diagnoses and their spectrum of CT appearances. At the same time the clinician should be confident that one of the presumptive diagnoses or the condition he wishes to exclude are detectable by CT in sufficient cases, and with sufficient specificity that CT scanning will contribute positively to patient care.

PATIENT POSITIONING

Early studies were virtually confined to transverse axial scanning, due to the construction of early machines which required a soft water-filled rubber bag to fit tightly around the cranial vault, the prime purpose being to overcome problems caused by the sudden transition from bone density to air density as the X-ray beam scanned across the head.

Modern machines have dispensed with the water bag, and now the use of general purpose machines with wide apertures, some incorporating tilting gantries, has freed the radiologist from many restrictions in patient positioning, and CT scanning has become considerably more versatile. The radiologist can exploit this freedom by varying the position of the patient at any time if a different projection may produce more useful information.

Even so a conventional starting point is required for cranial examinations, and this is usually related to the radiographic base line of the patient, which is a line between the external canthus of the eye and the external auditory meatus. The patient is positioned so that the plane of the scan slice is parallel to this line as indicated in Fig. 3.1a. From a starting point a little caudal to the base line the skull base to vertex can be covered in approximately ten adjacent slices. Flexing the patient's head on the neck creating an angle of about 10° between these planes permits a better 'view' of the contents of the posterior fossa. Coronal views may be taken by hyperextending the neck in the prone position, but this position may cause patient discomfort and therefore movement. It may be wise to accept a cut which is less than a true coronal section, but may convey equally useful information, rather than cause the patient such discomfort that scans may have to be repeated due to movement.

ENHANCEMENT WITH INTRAVENOUS IODINATED CONTRAST MEDIUM

At the time of writing there appear to be three general attitudes to this provocative question.

1. Perform plain scan, and enhance only when clinically or radiologically indicated.
2. Routine plain and enhanced scans.
3. Initial enhanced scan, subsequent plain scan if indicated.

A variety of factors may influence the decision by a department as to which philosophy they adopt, not least patient load and availability of medical supervision. On ethical grounds, the first approach appears to be the method of choice, as it avoids most unnecessary contrast injections and therefore minimizes the risk of morbidity and mortality from an injection of contrast medium which may generate no useful information.

However, this approach does require constant supervision of scans and also requires more skilled interpretation as lesions may be missed on plain scans and contrast injection omitted, although the lesion might have been obvious after enhancement. This method of supervision therefore calls for skilled supervision and an unwillingness to accept degraded scans, not infrequently necessitating repeat or overlapping slices.

Having shown an abnormality on plain scan, the necessity for contrast enhancement must be considered. In certain situations, it is well known that contrast injection will reveal no further information. A cerebral infarct with associated atrophy is unlikely to show pathological enhancement. However, a lesion consisting of low attenuation and swelling raises different possibilities; such a lesion may, for example, be ischaemic or neoplastic, and the pattern of enhancement may help the observer make this distinction. If, however, such a lesion is in a typical middle cerebral artery distribution and the history is strongly suggestive of an acute cerebral infarction, it is unlikely that further information will be gained from an enhanced scan. There is also the possibility that iodinated contrast medium further injures acutely ischaemic cerebral tissue. It is important that when the radiologist decides to administer contrast medium to a patient, he does so for justifiable and appropriate reasons. Each time iodinated contrast medium is injected, the patient is subjected to the risk of a potentially fatal reaction, and at the very least the discomfort of venepucture. If there is any doubt as to the indication for contrast injection, then discussion with the referring clinician is the simplest way to resolve it.

Situations in which a plain scan cannot be considered adequate fall into four main categories:

(a) Doubt about normality of plain scan
(b) Study of a technically difficult area, e.g. brain stem, posterior fossa, juxtasellar region.
(c) Suspicion of a lesion which may be isodense or too small to be seen before contrast injection, e.g. plaque of demyelination, AVM.
(d) Suspicion of a lesion known to cause subtle or inconclusive plain scan findings, but in which enhancement clarifies the picture, e.g. granulomatous meningitis.

METRIZAMIDE ENHANCEMENT OF THE CSF SPACES

A relatively small quantity of metrizamide injected into the sub-arachnoid space at lumbar puncture will diffuse through the CSF and allow CT examination of the cranial CSF spaces. Thus, masses encroaching on the basal cisterns may be detected as filling defects within the opacified cerebro-spinal fluid, e.g. acoustic neuroma encroaching on the cerebello-pontine angle cistern (Fig. 2.1), pituitary tumour extending into the chiasmatic cistern. Metrizamide may also be used to study the flow pattern of cerebro-spinal fluid. This may be of practical value in some patients in whom the distinction between atrophy and hydrocephalus cannot be definitely made.

XENON ENHANCEMENT

Xenon is an inert gas which is a safe anaesthetic when breathed in 70% mixture with oxygen. It is freely absorbed in body tissues, but is especially soluble in lipid and is taken up in the cerebral substance, particularly white matter, in sufficient concentration to increase the attenuation by up to 20 Hounsfield units. Lesions such as a demyelinating plaque (Fig. 2.2a,b), subdural haematoma or neoplasm frequently enhance less than the surrounding normal brain tissue and may be demonstrated more clearly, sometimes becoming evident only by this method of examination.

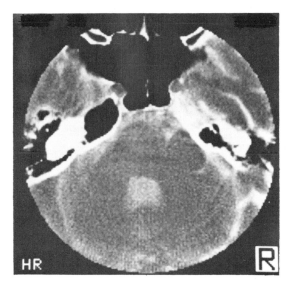

Fig. 2.1 Mass outlined in right cerebello-pontine angle. The brainstem is indented. Metrizamide enhanced CSF. Acoustic neuroma.

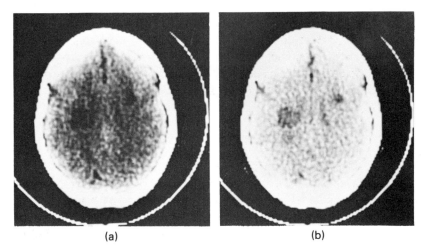

(a)   (b)

Fig. 2.2 (a, b) Scans before and after Xenon enhancement (taken at same window settings). The normal brain is seen to enhance; the lesions are more clearly seen with Xenon. Multiple sclerosis plaques.

CHAPTER THREE

Normal Anatomy

The interpretation of CT scans requires a sound knowledge of neuroanatomy. Precision in differential diagnosis depends both on the correct interpretation of CT attentuation changes and on an accurate determination of the site of a lesion in the brain and its effects on the surrounding structures.

A series of ten scans is displayed on pages 18–30 (Figs. 3.3 to 3.12) representing the 'routine' CT examination of the cranium.* The thickness of each scan slice shown here is 10 mm; the examination starts at the base of the skull, the plane being parallel to the orbito-meatal line, and extends up the cranium in a series of about ten slices. The relationship of the scan slices to the surface markings and to the cortex of the brain is shown in Figs. 3.1a and b, which also illustrate the boundaries of the lobes of the brain and the motor, sensory and visual cortices.

Figure 3.2 shows the relationship of the different named gyri and sulci to the scan slices.

Each scan slice is accompanied by three line drawings, illustrating different features of the scan. Figs. 3.3a to 3.12a illustrate the limits of the supra and infratentorial compartments and of the lobes of the brain. Figs. 3.3b to 3.12b illustrate the vascular territories of the brain. Figs. 3.3c to 3.12c show the course of the motor, sensory and visual tracts from their cortical connections, to the point where they leave the brain. The normal orbital scan is shown in Fig. 3.13.

---

* The scan pictures displayed show minor dilatation of the lateral ventricles and cortical sulci and are therefore not strictly normal, but serve better than normal scans for purposes of anatomical detail.

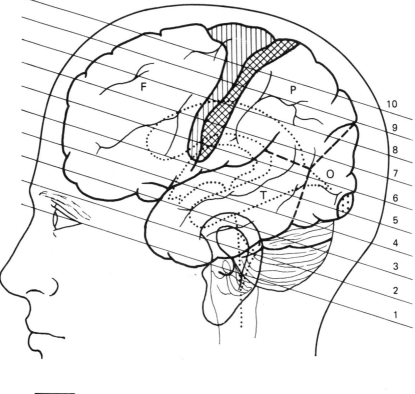

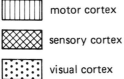
motor cortex

sensory cortex

visual cortex

Fig. 3.1a   Lateral view of head to show surface markings of orbito-meatal line, and the position of scan slices in relation to cerebral cortex. The ventricular system is outlined and the boundaries of the lobes and the motor, sensory and visual cortices are also shown.

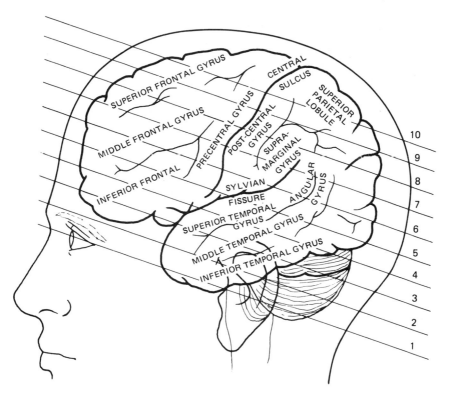

Fig. 3.1b   Lateral view of the head to show the relationship of the scan slices to the named gyri and sulci.

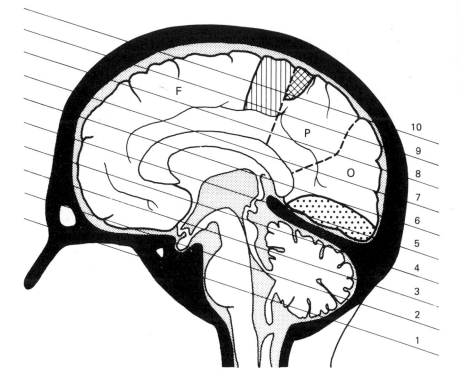

F = frontal

P = parietal

O = occipital

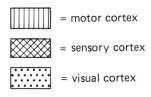 = motor cortex

= sensory cortex

= visual cortex

Fig. 3.2a   Midline sagittal section showing the relation of the scan slices to the medial aspect of the cerebral cortex, the third ventricle and the posterior fossa. The boundaries of the lobes and the motor, sensory and visual cortices are shown.

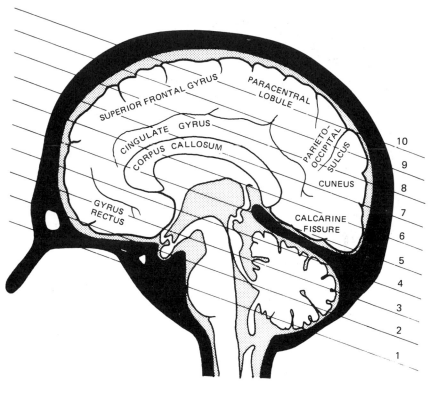

Fig. 3.2b Midline sagittal section showing named sulci and gyri.

Scan Section 1: Along the orbito-meatal line

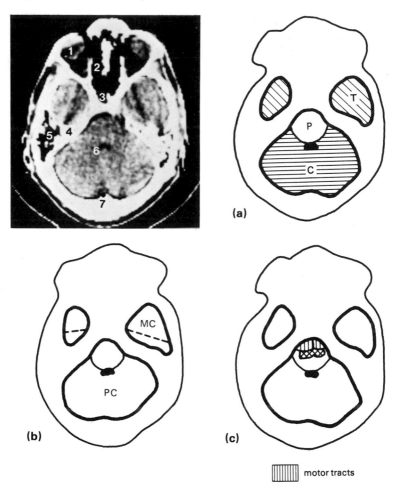

Fig. 3.3

1. Left globe.
2. Ethmoid sinus.
3. Sphenoid sinus.
4. Petrous ridge.
5. Mastoid air cells.
6. Fourth ventricle.
7. Internal occipital protuberance, and upper limit of cisterna magna.

(a) T – Anterior part of temporal lobe in middle fossa.   P – Pons.
C – Cerebullum.

(b) The poles and superolateral parts of the temporal lobes are usually supplied by the middle cerebral arteries, the posterior cerebral artery supplying the remainder.

(c) The motor (pyramidal) and sensory tracts (medial lemniscus) are situated in the anterior part of the pons.

Scan Section 2: 10 mm above the orbito-meatal line

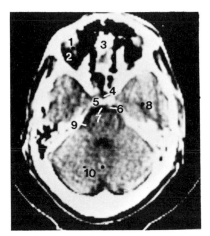

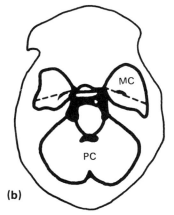

(a)

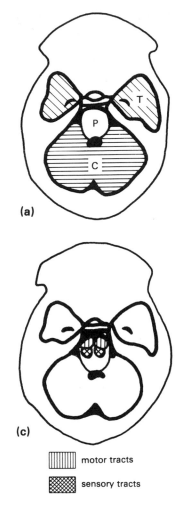

(b)

(c)

▨▨▨ motor tracts

▨▨▨ sensory tracts

Fig. 3.4

1. Optic nerve.
2. Orbital fat.
3. Cribriform plate of ethmoid bone.
4. Pituitary fossa.
5. Dorsum sellae.
6. Basilar artery.
7. Pontine cistern.
8. Temporal horn of lateral ventricle.
9. Cerebellopontine angle.
10. Vermis of cerebellum.

(a) T – Temporal lobe   P – Pons   C – Cerebellum
(b) The boundary between the middle and posterior cerebral territories is shown.
(c) The motor and sensory tracts are situated anteriorly in the brain stem.

Scan Section 3: 20 mm above the orbito-meatal line

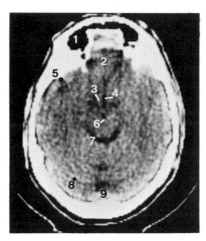

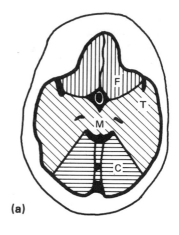

(a)

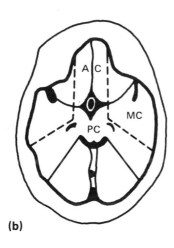

(b)

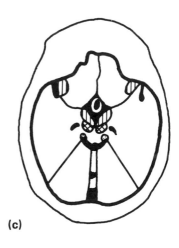

(c)

Fig. 3.5

1. Frontal sinus.
2. Gyri recti.
3. Hypothalamus in chiasmatic cistern.
4. Third ventricle-anterior part.

5. Sylvian Fissure.
6. Interpeduncular fossa.
7. Quadrigeminal cistern.
8. Cerebellar sulcus.
9. Cisterna Magna.

(a) F − Frontal lobe.
   T − Temporal lobe.
   C − Cerebellum.
   M − Midbrain.

The posterior limits of the frontal lobes are shown extending lateral to the chiasmatic cistern. The tentorial edge, is also shown. The chiasmatic cistern contains the anterior recesses of the third ventricle and hypothalamus.

(b) Three vascular territories are outlined corresponding to the anterior middle and posterior cerebral territories.

(c) In addition to the motor and sensory tracts in the midbrain the origin of the visual tract is seen from the lateral geniculate body. The lowermost extent of the motor cortex is shown in the frontal lobe adjacent to the anterior limit of the Sylvian fissure.

Scan Section 4: 30 mm above the orbito-meatal line

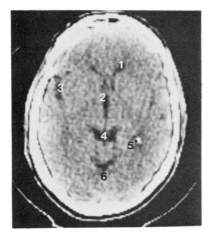

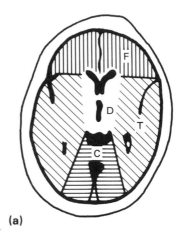

(a)

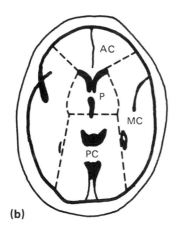

(b)

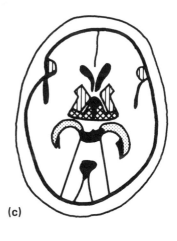

(c)

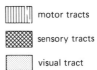

▦ motor tracts	
▨ sensory tracts	
▧ visual tract	

Scan Section 4: 30 mm above the orbito-meatal line

Fig. 3.6

1. Frontal horn of lateral ventricle.
2. Third ventricle.
3. Sylvian Fissure.
4. Quadrigeminal bodies and cistern.
5. Choroid plexus in trigone of lateral ventricle
6. Superior cerebellar cistern.

(a) F — Frontal lobe.
   D — Diencephalon (thalamus and basal nuclei).
   T — Temporal lobe.
   C — Cerebellum.

(b) In addition to the anterior middle and posterior cerebral territories shown here, the diencephalon and internal capsular region is shown to be supplied by perforating arteries which arise from the terminal internal carotid and proximal anterior and middle cerebral trunks. The posterior cerebral supply includes the thalamus.

(c) Three tracts are again outlined in this diagram. The ascending motor fibres constitute the internal capsule at this level and are illustrated by the angulated hatched area lateral to the thalami. The thalamus is the main sensory nucleus and it is connected to the posterior limb of the internal capsule as shown. The optic radiation is shown passing back towards the occipital lobe.

Scan Section 5: 40 mm above the orbito-meatal line

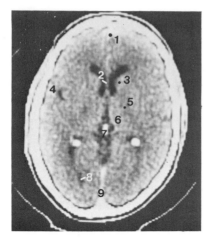
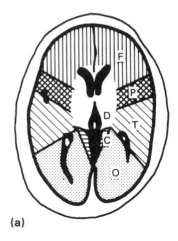

(a)

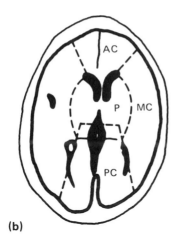

(b)

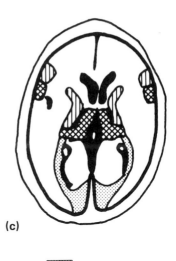

(c)

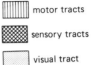

motor tracts

sensory tracts

visual tract

Scan Section 5: 40 mm above the orbito-meatal line

Fig. 3.7

1. Falx cerebri.
2. Interventricular septum (septum pellucidum)
3. Head of caudate nucleus.
4. Sylvian Fissure.
5. Internal Capsule.
6. Thalamus.
7. Calcified pineal gland
8. Occipital horn of the lateral ventricle.
9. Straight sinus in falx.

(a) F — Frontal lobe   O — Occipital lobe
     P — Parietal lobe   D — Diencephalon
     T — Temporal lobe   C — Apex of posterior fossa.

(b) The vascular territories are similar to the subjacent scan. The middle cerebral artery has the most extensive area of supply.

(c) The internal capsule is demonstrated lateral to the thalamus. The thalamus is connected to the sensory tracts in the posterior limb of the internal capsule, and the optic radiation fibres sweep around through the temporal lobe to the occipital cortex. The lower end of the pre- and post-central gyri are shown.

Scan Section 6: 50 mm above the orbito-meatal line

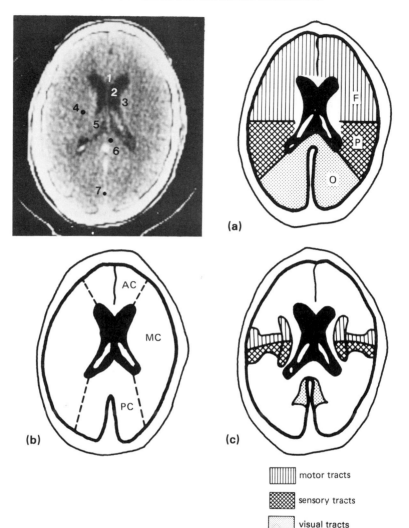

(a)

(b)

(c)

motor tracts

sensory tracts

visual tracts

Fig. 3.8
1. Body of corpus callosum.
2. Body of the lateral ventricle.
3. Body of the caudate nucleus.
4. Corona radiata
5. Choroid plexus.
6. Splenium of the corpus callosum.
7. Falx cerebri.

(a) F – Frontal lobe. P – Parietal lobe. O – Occipital lobe.

(b) Only three vascular territories are seen at this level.

(c) At this level the motor and sensory fibres in the corona radiata extend laterally to reach their cortical projections. The most superior part of the visual cortex is still visible.

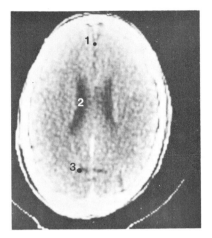
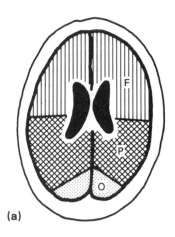

(a)

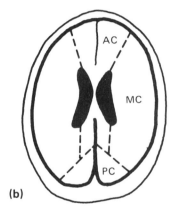

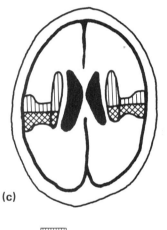

(b)

(c)

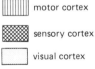

motor cortex

sensory cortex

visual cortex

Fig. 3.9
1. Falx and interhemispheric fissure.
2. Lateral ventricles.
3. Parieto-occipital sulcus.
(a) F – Frontal. P – Parietal. O – Occipital.
(b) The anterior cerebral artery territory can be seen to extend back to the territory of the posterior cerebral artery.
(c) The motor and sensory radiations are again shown.

Scan Section 8: 70 mm above the orbito-meatal line

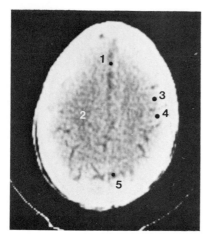

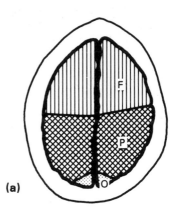

(a)

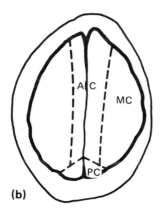

(b)

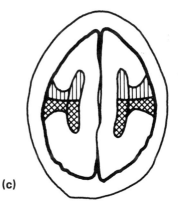

(c)

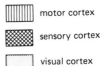

	motor cortex
	sensory cortex
	visual cortex

Fig. 3.10

1. Interhemispheric fissure and falx.
2. Corona radiata.
3. Pre-central gyrus.
4. Post-central gyrus.
5. Parieto-occipital fissure.

(a) F – Frontal lobe. P – Parietal lobe. O – Occipital lobe.
(b) Vascular territories are similar to the subjacent scan.
(c) The motor and sensory radiations are still seen.

Scan Section 9: 80 mm above the orbito-meatal line

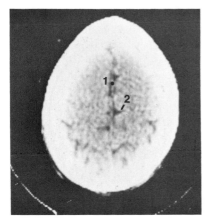

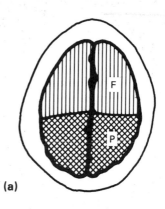

(a)

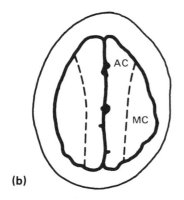

(b)

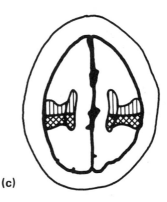

(c)

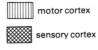

motor cortex

sensory cortex

Fig. 3.11
1. Falx cerebri
2. Cingulate sulcus
(a) F — Frontal lobe. P — Parietal lobe.
(b) The anterior cerebral artery territory extends throughout the length of the scan flanked laterally by the middle cerebral artery territories.
(c) The motor and sensory radiations are shown.

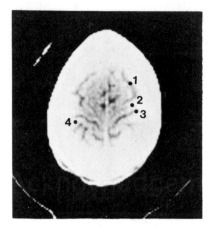
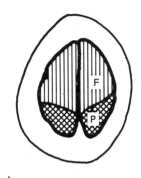

(a)

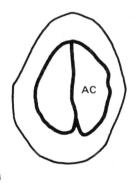

(b)

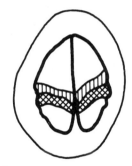

(c)

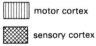 motor cortex

sensory cortex

Fig. 3.12
1. Superior frontal sulcus.
2. Pre-central gyrus.
3. Central sulcus (Rolandic fissure).
4. Post-central gyrus.
(a) F – Frontal lobe. P – Parietal lobe.
(b) Cerebral tissue here is supplied by the anterior cerebral artery.
(c) The motor and sensory cortices are situated in pre- and post-central gyri.

Normal Orbital Scan

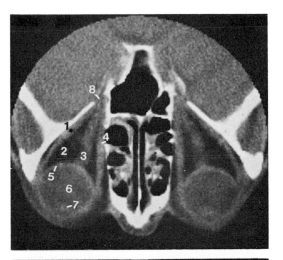

(a)

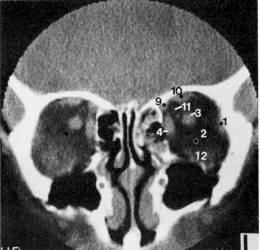

(b)

Fig. 3.13

(a) Axial scan
1. Lateral rectus muscle.
2. Orbital fat.
3. Optic nerve.
4. Medial rectus muscle.
5. Sclera.
6. Vitreous humor.
7. Lens.
8. Superior orbital fissure.

(b) Coronal
1. Lateral rectus muscle.
2. Orbital fat.
3. Optic nerve.
4. Medial rectus muscle.
9. Superior oblique muscle.
10. Superior rectus muscle.
11. Nasociliary nerve.
12. Inferior rectus muscle.

CHAPTER FOUR

How to Report a Scan

The abnormal features seen on a CT scan may be described in the following terms which can be used as a basis for reporting a scan:

1. abnormal tissue attenuation
2. mass effect
3. loss of tissue
4. site of lesion
5. characteristics of contrast enhancement.

1. Abnormal Tissue Attenuation

Note the areas of abnormal attenuation. The abnormalities may be described in the following terms:

(a) size	– extensive, large, small
(b) shape	– rounded, wedge-shaped, linear
(c) margin	– clearly defined, irregular, poorly defined
(d) attenuation	– high – should be measured ? blood ? calcium
	– low – measurement may indicate CSF, fat
	– mixed
	– brain (isodense)

The abnormality frequently consists of the lesion itself and a tissue reaction in the form of oedema. If the distinction is evident, from the outset, or after contrast injection, then the description should indicate this, rather than use vague descriptions such as mixed attenuation area when one is describing a high attenuation lesion with surrounding oedema.

2. Mass effect

Note presence of mass effect. This can be described as follows:

(a) mild, moderate, marked, as indicated by midline shift, ventricular compression, effacement of cortical sulci
(b) presence of transtentorial herniation

(c) whether the degree of mass effect is in proportion to the size of the lesion indicated by abnormal attenuation.

Not infrequently, the descriptive portion of a CT report will describe the lesion as having no mass effect, and is followed by a diagnosis of a mass lesion. Such obvious contradictions should be avoided by employing descriptive phrases such as 'no apparent mass effect'.

When describing a large mass lesion, it is unnecessary to describe the entire evidence of mass effect such as sulcal effacement, cistern encroachment, ventricular compression, etc, etc; such features should be described concisely but a comment on specific features such as contralateral ventricular dilatation or obvious brain stem compression is more helpful.

3. Loss of Tissue

Note the size of:

(a) the ventricles
(b) cerebral and cerebellar sulci
(c) sylvian and interhemispheric fissures
(d) basal cisterns.

One should resist the temptation to automatically describe a lesion of low attenuation with associated atrophy as an infarct. Sometimes the non-specific expression of 'focal brain damage' is more accurate.

4. Site of Lesion

The following anatomical distinctions should be made:

(a) supratentorial or infratentorial
(b) frontal, temporal, occipital or parietal, or a combination of these
(c) brainstem or cerebellum
(d) a more detailed anatomical site may be specified (e.g. internal capsule).

Mass lesions frequently result in considerable distortion of normal anatomy. This may result in, for example, a temporal lobe tumour, extending into the high parietal region. Description of such lesions should take this into account and describe where possible the primary site of a lesion with its extensions, rather than a vague description of a tempero-parietal mass, which would not indicate the relationship of the mass to the sylvian fissure.

Distortion of normal structures must always be taken into consideration as failure to do so will lead to an overestimate of the extent of a lesion.

5. Characteristics of Contrast Enhancement

The pattern of contrast enhancement may be described as follows:

(a) degree   – slight, moderate, dense

(b) configuration   – patchy, homogeneous, ring, linear, serpiginous.

It is of paramount importance to bear the partial volume effect in mind in all considerations of attenuation characteristics, including situations involving enhancing lesions. Similarly, slight change in angle or plane of section will exert considerable influence on these features. Where there is doubt, the use of phrases such as questionable or equivocal are perfectly valid, and likely to induce less error than saying definitely one way or another when such a distinction is not possible from the available evidence.

Conclusion

If the report is long the main features should be summarized succinctly, ideally in one sentence. A diagnosis or short differential diagnosis should be offered.

CHAPTER FIVE

Detection of Pathology by CT Scan

CT appearances may be classified according to their specificity in diagnosis in the following ways:

(a) Pathognomic.
(b) Strongly suggestive of a particular diagnosis.
(c) Abnormal but non-specific.

In addition the scan may be:

(d) Normal.

The value of CT as a screening procedure must not be underestimated. A normal scan will exclude certain diagnostic possibilities, although it must be remembered that there will be phases in the natural history of most lesions when the CT scan will be normal.

It is important to acquire a working knowledge of the potential contribution of CT scanning to specific diagnostic possibilities whether the scan is normal or abnormal. The following lists are based on the authors experience and are necessarily dogmatic. The classification has been restricted to what are considered the three most useful categories. The incidence of each category in the context of a particular diagnosis is graded as follows:

+ + + = predominantly
+ + = frequently
+ = occasionally

LESION	Degree of specificity of scan appearance		
	Strongly suggestive of diagnosis	*Abnormal but non-specific*	*Normal*
1. Congenital			
Leukodystrophy	+ +	+ +	+
Neurofibromatosis	+	+	+ +
Tuberose sclerosis	+ + +	+	+
Sturge-Weber syndrome	+ +	+	+
Von-Hippel Lindau syndrome	+	+ +	+

Comment: The subependymal nodules of tuberose sclerosis are virtually pathognomonic.

2. Trauma			
Intracerebral haematoma	+ + +	+	+
Subdural haematoma	+ +	+	+
Contusion	+ +	+	+
Extradural haematoma	+ + +	+	+
Subarachnoid haemorrhage	+ +	+	+

3. Tumours: Malignant			
'Glioma'	+ +	+ +	+
Metastasis	+	+ +	+
Carcinomatous meningitis	+	+	+ +
Medulloblastoma	+	+ +	+
Haemangioblastoma	+	+ +	+
Pineal region tumour	+ + +	+	+
Chordoma	+	+ +	+
Microglioma	+	+ + +	+

Comment: A pineal region tumour with fat, calcium and soft tissue densities is virtually pathognomic of teratoma.

Tumours: Benign			
Meningioma	+ +	+ +	+
Pituitary adenoma	+ +	+ +	+
Craniopharyngioma	+ +	+ +	+
Acoustic neuroma	+ + +	+	+
Colloid cyst of 3rd ventricle	+ + +	+	+
Choroid plexus papilloma	+ +	+	+

LESION	Degree of specificity of scan appearance		
	Strongly suggestive of diagnosis	*Abnormal but non-specific*	*Normal*
4. Inflammatory			
Acute pyogenic meningitis	−	−	+ + +
Abscess	+ +	+ +	+
Chronic granulomatous meningitis (TB, sarcoidosis, fungus)	+	+	+ +
Herpes simplex encephalitis	+ +	+ +	+
Progressive multifocal leukoencephalopathy	+	+ +	+

Comment: No scan abnormality in uncomplicated acute pyogenic meningitis.

5. Vascular			
Intracerebral haemorrhage	+ + +	+	+
Subarachnoid haemorrhage	+ +	+	+
Aneurysm	+	+	+ + +
Angioma	+ +	+	+
Cerebral infarct	+ +	+ +	+
Posterior fossa infarct	+	+	+ +
Sagittal sinus thrombosis	+	+ +	+ +
Hypertensive encephalopathy	+	+	+ +
Multi-infarct dementia	+ +	+ +	+

Comment: A dural angioma is not usually detected by CT.

6. Degenerative disorders			
Parkinson's disease	+	+ +	+ +
Huntington's chorea	+	+ +	+ +
Wilson's disease	+	+ +	+ +

Comment: The conditions above usually show non-specific atrophic change. Alzheimer's disease is a very frequent cause of atrophy, but shows no specific CT features.

LESION	Degree of specificity of scan appearance		
	Strongly suggestive of diagnosis	*Abnormal but non-specific*	*Normal*
7. Toxic and Metabolic			
Chronic alcoholism	−	+ + +	+
Carbon monoxide poisoning	−	+ +	+ +
Radionecrosis	+	+ + +	+
Hepatic/Renal failure	−	+ +	+ +
Disseminated necrotising leukoencephalopathy	+	+ +	+
8. Parasitic			
Hydatid disease	+ + +	−	−
Cysticercosis	+	+ +	+
9. Others			
Hydrocephalus	+ + +	+	−
Multiple sclerosis	+	+ +	+ +

CHAPTER SIX

Differential Diagnosis

(A) ELEMENTS OF DIAGNOSIS

The presence of an intracranial lesion may be inferred from any one of three features demonstrated by CT scan.

1. Loss of tissue.
2. Mass effect.
3. Abnormal tissue attenuation.

Further interpretation of the scan then involves accurate anatomical analysis so that the site of each lesion is determined. In addition the pattern of any enhancement of the lesion after intravenous contrast administration is frequently very helpful in differential diagnosis, often provides essential information, is sometimes virtually pathognomic, and occasionally is the only method of demonstrating any abnormality. To (1), (2) and (3) therefore, we may add

4. Anatomical siting of lesion(s).
5. Characteristics of contrast enhancement.

After consideration of these five fundamental features, a radiological differential diagnosis may be reached, and considered in the clinical context.

(1) Loss of Tissue

This is frequently obvious and seen as thinning or cavitation of the cerebral substance either focally or diffusely. Its presence may also be inferred from widened CSF spaces, indicated by ventricular dilation or subarachnoid widening, either of which may be focal or diffuse (Fig. 6.1). Loss of tissue is the common end-point of many pathological processes, e.g. haemorrhage, infarction, demyelination.

If tissue loss is sufficiently longstanding there may be associated changes in the skull vault or base. The finding of slight lateral ventricular asymmetry is within normal limits.

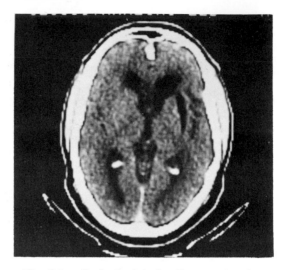

Fig. 6.1   Cavity in right lentiform region due to previous haemorrhage. Widened Sylvian fissure and dilated right frontal horn are evidence of atrophy.

(2) Mass Effect

Evidence is seen in the form of distorted CSF spaces, usually the ventricular system, less obviously the subarachnoid space and its cisterns. Obstruction of the ventricular system or subarachnoid space is a frequent end result of such distortion.

The spectrum of distortion of the CSF spaces ranges from gross lateral ventricular hydrocephalus due, for example, to a tumour obliterating the third ventricle, to subtle effacement of cerebral sulci from an underlying swelling. An appropriately placed mass may obstruct and loculate parts of the ventricular system, for example a temporal tumour not infrequently obstructs the temporal horn (Fig. 6.2). A hemisphere mass may cause dilation of the contralateral ventricle by kinking and obstruction of the foramen of Munro (Fig. 6.3). Uncal herniation is detected by observing distortion or obliteration of the chiasmatic cistern. On occasion anatomical distortion can lead to an overestimate of the extent of a mass; for example a deep hemisphere tumour may so displace the basal ganglia and thalamus that the distorted anatomy may simulate an extension of the tumour (Fig. 6.4), and perhaps lead to the erroneous impression of an intraventricular component. The mass effect of certain lesions is increased by coexisting oedema. If the lesion is of low attenuation, then the mass and its oedema may merge imperceptibly. In the absence of contrast enhancement the distinction is difficult.

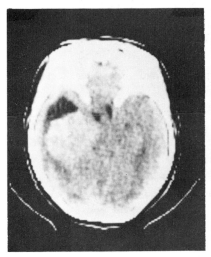

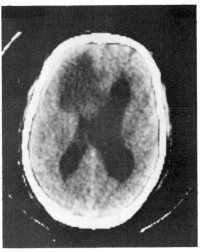

Fig. 6.2 Intraventricular meningioma obstructing the left temporal horn.

Fig. 6.3 Left frontal glioma causing contralateral hydrocephalus.

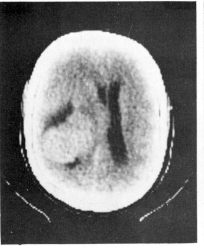

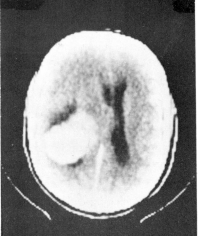

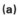

(a)

(b)

Fig. 6.4 (a) Left hemisphere tumour apparently extending into the lateral ventricle.
(b) Contrast injection reveals true extent of tumour. The intraventricular mass is due to displaced thalamus.

(3) Abnormal Tissue Attenuation

It is most convenient to describe abnormal cerebral tissue attenuation in relation to that of normal cerebral substance. Lesions having the same visual density as cerebral substance are referred to as isodense with brain. Tissues differing from cerebral attenuation are referred to as high or low attenuation areas, or as being hyper- or hypodense.

Tissue of attenuation more than 50 Hounsfield units suggests calcification or haemorrhage, although some lesions may occasionally appear significantly hyperdense without either of these features histologically, e.g. colloid cyst. Measurement of tissue attenuation can be helpful, although partial volume effect may distort the attenuation value of a structure. Intracerebral haemorrhage may occasionally reach an attenuation value greater than 90 HU; but if the lesion measures much more than this simple haemorrhage can be excluded. If a low density lesion has negative values in the region of −100 HU then fatty tissue is present and a compatible diagnosis such as dermoid or lipoma can be suggested (Fig. 6.5).

The attenuation values must be appropriate before certain diagnoses may be entertained. For example, lesions containing blood, such as an angiomatous malformation or aneurysm, owe their attenuation to the blood they contain; the lesion should therefore be slightly hyperdense prior to contrast injection. A porencephalic cyst by definition contains CSF and therefore an inappropriate attenuation value excludes the diagnosis or indicates a complication such as haemorrhage. Conversely, low attenuation

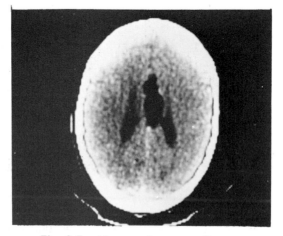

Fig. 6.5   Lipoma of corpus callosum.

lesions are unlikely to contain florid pathological circulation although enhancement may occur in these lesions due to blood brain barrier breakdown.

Low attenuation, non-enhancing sharply circumscribed lesions suggest cysts, but the only absolute indication of a cystic lesion is the uncommon sign of layering either of contrast medium (Fig. 6.6a,b) or sediment within the lesion, prior to contrast enhancement. Cystic lesions are not necessarily of very low attenuation; the contents of the cyst determine precise values.

Enhancement of a lesion following injection of contrast medium may be due either to extravasation from breakdown of the 'blood-brain barrier' or to the inherent vascularity of a lesion. If enhancement is due to the latter it will cease as soon as the contrast is excreted, and the intensity of enhancement therefore depends very much on the timing of the scan. If it is due to the former it will persist for longer after the injection, and the pattern of enhancement may alter with time due to diffusion of the contrast medium. The enhancement of many lesions is due to a summation of both mechanisms, but also depends on the quantity of contrast medium administered.

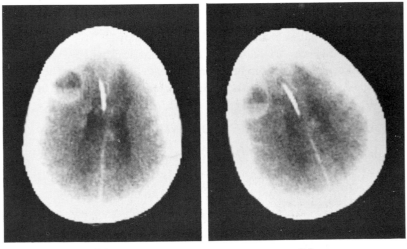

(a)   **(b)**

Fig. 6.6 (a, b)   Enhanced scans of a cystic tumour showing layering of contrast medium within the cyst; confirmed by tilting the patient's head.

(B) SYSTEM OF DIFFERENTIAL DIAGNOSES

The following system depends on the presence or absence of three fundamental features on the **unenhanced** scan: abnormality in attenuation, mass effect, and tissue loss. Having inspected the scan, the viewer must decide which combination of the features is present.

1. Abnormal attenuation with mass effect.
2. Abnormal attenuation without mass effect.
3. Abnormal attenuation with tissue loss.
4. Normal attenuation with mass effect.
5. Normal attenuation without mass effect (i.e. normal scan).
6. Normal attenuation with tissue loss.

Three common plain scan findings are:

7. Multiple lesions.
8. Calcified lesions.
9. Low attenuation in the white matter.

Distinctive patterns of enhancement include:

10. Lesions showing dense enhancement.
11. Lesions showing ring enhancement.

Lists intended as aids in differential diagnosis and arranged according to the scan observations enumerated above now follow.

The lists are necessarily dogmatic and cannot be exhaustive but give an indication of the main differential diagnosis in each situation. The lesions are discussed in more detail elsewhere and cross reference should be made freely.

1. ABNORMAL ATTENUATION WITH MASS EFFECT

(a) **Low Attenuation**
Well circumscribed
    Arachnoid cyst
    Porencephaly
    Occasional glioma
    Dermoid, epidermoid
    Hydatid cyst

Less sharply circumscribed (frequently because of associated oedema)

    Recent infarct
    Resolving haemorrhage
    Tumour – glioma
          – metastasis
          – microglioma
          – rarely meningioma
    Abscess
    Venous thrombosis
    Encephalitis

(b) Mixed attenuation

    Tumour – glioma
          – metastasis
          – meningioma
          – haemangioblastoma
          – dermoid/teratoma
          – craniopharyngioma
          – pinealoma
    Abscess
    Haemorrhagic infarct
    Haemorrhagic contusion
    Hamartoma

(c) Raised attenuation

    Tumour – meningioma
          – metastasis
          – microglioma
          – glioma
          – medulloblastoma
          – pinealoma
    Craniopharyngioma
    Colloid cyst
    Haematoma
    Large aneurysm–AVM
    Chordoma

2. ABNORMAL ATTENUATION WITH NO MASS EFFECT

Infiltrating or small tumour
Angiomatous malformation
Infarct/porencephaly
Encephalitis
Venous occlusion
Leukodystrophy
Progressive multifocal leukoencephalopathy
Necrotizing leukoencephalopathy
Granulomatous/neoplastic meningitis
Subarachnoid haemorrhage
Intraventricular haemorrhage

3. ABNORMAL ATTENUATION WITH LOSS OF TISSUE

Mature infarct
Porencephaly
Post-haemorrhagic cavity
Post-encephalitic (herpes especially)
Post-traumatic including surgical
Radiotherapy
Basal ganglia cavitation – anoxia
                              – Parkinsonism
                              – Wilson's disease

4. NORMAL ATTENUATION WITH MASS EFFECT

Isodense swelling: trauma, inflammatory, postoperative
Acute infarct
Subdural collection – 7–20 days old
Resolving haemorrhage
Occasional tumour – glioma, meningioma
Hydrocephalus

5. **NORMAL ATTENUATION WITH NO MASS EFFECT** (compatible with normal unenhanced scan)

    Acute cerebral, cerebellar or brainstem infarction
    Angiomatous malformation
    Mutiple sclerosis
    Venous thrombosis
    Subarachnoid haemorrhage

6. **NORMAL ATTENUATION WITH TISSUE LOSS**

    Diffuse atrophy – cerebral, cerebellar or brainstem

7. **MULTIPLE LESIONS**

    Tumour – metastases
            – microglioma
            – occasionally glioma, meningioma
    Inflammatory – abscesses
                  – granulomata – tuberculous
                                – sarcoid
                                – fungal
    Multiple sclerosis
    Infarcts
    Multifocal haemorrhage – trauma, malignant hypertension
                                    – blood dyscrasia
    Tuberose sclerosis
    Toxoplasmosis
    Cysticerosis
    Basal ganglia calcification

8. CALCIFIED LESIONS

Craniopharyngioma
Astrocytoma
Oligodendroglioma
Ependymoma
Pinealoma
Meningioma
Metastasis (rarely)
AVM
Tuberose sclerosis
Hamartoma
Cysticerosis
Toxoplasmosis
Idiopathic (brain stone)
Chronic subdural haematoma $\Big\}$ rarely
Old intracebrebral haematoma
Atheromatous vessels, aneurysms
Normal
Pineal
Choroid plexus
Basal ganglia
dura

9. LOW ATTENUATION IN THE WHITE MATTER

Oedema (of any cause)
Tumour extension through white matter
Encephalitis
Trauma
Periventricular lucency in hydrocephalus
Binswanger's disease
Radionecrosis
Renal/hepatic failure
Leukoencephalopathy
Leukodystrophy

10. LESIONS SHOWING DENSE HOMOGENEOUS ENHANCEMENT

Meningioma
Aneurysm
Ependymoma
Metastasis
Choroid plexus papilloma
Glioma (occasionally)
Arteriovenous malformation
Acute infarct (unusually)

11. LESIONS SHOWING RING ENHANCEMENT

Abscess
Glioma
Metastasis
Acute infarct (occasionally)
Resolving haemorrhage
Craniopharyngioma (occasionally)
Pituitary tumour (unusually)
Giant, partly thrombosed, aneurysm

Synopsis to Chapter Seven

CONGENITAL
Malformation
   Agenesis of corpus callosum
   Lipoma of corpus callosum
Leukodystrophy
Phakomatoses
   Neurofibromatosis
   Tuberose Sclerosis
   Sturge–Weber syndrome
   Von Hippel–Lindau syndrome

TRAUMA
Haemorrhage
Contusion
Swelling

TUMOUR
Glioma
Metastasis
Microglioma
Pineal region tumours

INFLAMMATORY
Abscess (pyogenic, tuberculous)
Encephalitis
Progressive multifocal leukoencephalopathy

VASCULAR
Intracerebral haemorrhage
Infarction
Venous Occlusion

DEGENERATIVE

TOXIC AND METABOLIC

PARASITIC

MULTIPLE SCLEROSIS

CHAPTER SEVEN

The Cerebrum

CONGENITAL

Malformation

1. Agenesis of corpus callosum. CT shows widely separated lateral ventricles with the third ventricle lying high between them. There is frequently, dilatation of the trigones, and in particular occipital horns.
2. Lipoma of corpus callosum. CT shows irregular mass of fat attenuation in the region of the corpus callosum (Fig. 6.5).

Leukodystrophy is the generic term for a group of conditions, usually inherited in an autosomal recessive manner, in which the grey matter is relatively spared but progressive bilateral white matter degeneration occurs, sometimes leading to considerable atrophy. The CT manifestation of this is abnormally low attenuation of the cerebral white matter, as well as evidence of tissue loss.

Phakomatoses (also called the neuro-ectodermal dysplasias) are hereditary disorders often manifesting in childhood. There are four relatively common disorders in this group:

1. Neurofibromatosis (Fig. 7.1)

Dysplasia — skull
            — brain, e.g. hemiatrophy, heterotopia
            — orbits and contents
Neoplasm — cranial nerve sheath (acoustic neuroma, optic nerve sheath meningioma)
            — optic nerve glioma (may be bilateral)
            — glioma
            — ependymona
            — meningioma

A neoplasm occurs in about 5% of cases; choroid plexus hypertrophy may be seen.

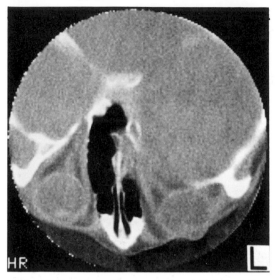

Fig. 7.1 Neurofibromatosis: deficient left sphenoid wing with encroachment of contents of an enlarged middle fossa on the orbit.

2. Tuberose Sclerosis (Fig. 7.2)

Paraventricular masses – often multiple, calcified.

Dilated ventricles.

Tendency for enlarging tumours, typically giant cell astrocytoma, to develop near foramen of Munro and lead to obstructive hydrocephalus.

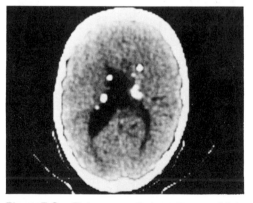

Fig. 7.2 Tuberose Sclerosis: multiple paraventricular calcifications.

3. Sturge-Weber Syndrome (Fig. 7.3)

Cortical calcification — gyriform pattern not evident on CT
                 — CT much more sensitive than conventional radiography

Hemiatrophy   — of skull and brain with subarachmoid space widening on side of lesion.

The CT lesion is usually clinically associated with a facial naevus. There is no intracranial angiomatous malformation, but the affected brain may show some enhancement.

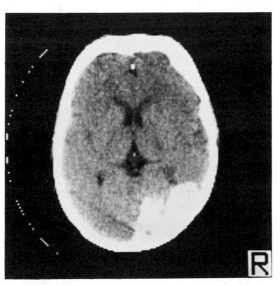

Fig. 7.3 Sturge-Weber Syndrome: typical calcification in right posterior temporal and occipital regions. The lesion has no mass effect.

4. Von Hippel — Lindau Syndrome

Multiple cerebellar haemangioblastomas associated with a retinal lesion. The cerebellar lesions are often low attenuation cysts with mural nodules which enhance. They may be very small and multiple and occasionally supratentorial.

TRAUMA

The following patterns may be seen:

1. Focal high attenuation haemorr-
   hage with mass effect   — intracerebral
                                              — subdural
                                              — subarachnoid
                                              — extradural
2. Mixed attenuation with mass effect: — haemorrhagic contusion
3. Reduced attenuation with mass
   effect: — contusion
4. Brain attenuation with mass effect: — isodense brain swelling
                                              (contusion)
5. Skull Fracture

Extradural and subdural haematomas are usually associated with trauma; they are discussed with subarachnoid haemorrhage in Chapter 9.

A typical intracerebral haemorrhage can be diagnosed without difficulty. An area of blood attenuation is demonstrated, usually with a surrounding rim of low attenuation, and associated with a variable amount of mass effect. Sometimes it is not clear from the history, however, whether the lesion is traumatic or spontaneous — in general a traumatic haemorrhage is associated with rather more peripheral low attenuation and in addition there is frequently evidence of more diffuse brain swelling.

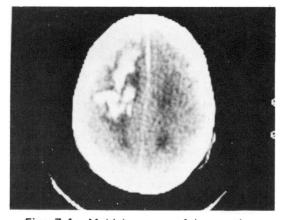

Fig. 7.4 Multiple areas of haemorrhage within low attenuation region. Haemorrhagic contusion.

The scan may yield further information such as the presence of skull fracture, subarachnoid or intraventricular bleeding.

Cerebral contusion appears as a low attenuation area or areas associated with brain swelling. It may be haemorrhagic, and it then has the added feature of areas of high (blood) attenuation, usually multifocal (Fig. 7.4). Brain swelling frequently follows trauma, it may be of low attenuation or isodense. Pathologically it may be due to contusion of the brain, or to shearing of the white matter tracts, when CT may demonstrate low attenuation in the white matter. Isodense swelling may only be appreciated in retrospect, when the ventricles and sulci return to normal size as the swelling resolves. A frequent end result of trauma is destruction of cerebral substance which may be seen focally as an area of low attenuation, or as more diffuse atrophy indicated by dilatation of the adjacent CSF spaces.

TUMOURS

The following chart indicates the steps involved in diagnosing an *intracerebral tumour* from CT evidence of an *intracranial mass*.

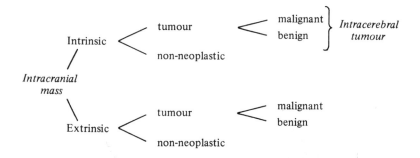

An intrinsic tumour arises within the brain (e.g. glioma) whereas an extrinsic tumour arises outside the brain (e.g. convexity meningioma). Intrinsic tumours are usually malignant and extrinsic tumours are usually benign, at least in some senses of these words; malignancy here meaning the actual infiltrative invasion of brain tissue. In the majority of cases of intracranial tumour, the diagnosis lies between a malignant intrinsic tumour and a benign extrinsic tumour burrowing into the cerebral substance.

Non-neoplastic lesions most likely to result in erroneous diagnosis as a tumour are recent infarcts, angiomatous malformation, abscess or granuloma, enhancing multiple sclerosis plaques, resolving haemorrhage, radionecrosis and inflammation.

1. Glioma

The CT spectrum of glioma is wide. Typically, a mass of mixed high and low attenuation is seen, with peripheral low attenuation often extending into the white matter tracts creating the familiar appearance of 'fingers' of oedema (Fig. 7.5). Calcification may be present, and this has some correlation with relatively low malignancy, but this is not an absolute criterion. Histological study frequently shows that the degree of malignancy of a

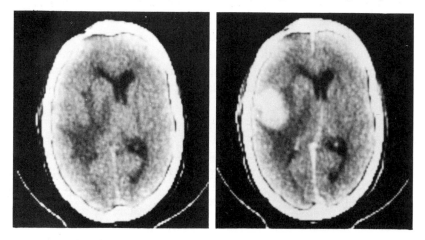

Fig. 7.5 (a, b)   Irregular low attenuation (oedema) associated with a tumour (glioma) which is only revealed by contrast injection.

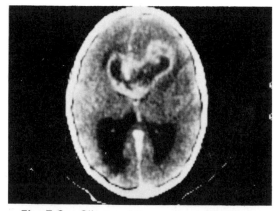

Fig. 7.6   Glioma of the corpus callosum extending across the midline with dilatation of the posterior parts of the lateral ventricles. Enhanced scan.

glioma may vary markedly within the same tumour mass, but in general the more benign elements are low attenuation areas on the scan, often contain calcium, and show virtually no enhancement, whereas the malignant component may show marked enhancement. Oedema around a glioma is variable; its absence is unusual but does not exclude the diagnosis. However, peripheral low attenuation in relation to a glioma is not necessarily oedema and infiltration of the white matter by glioma tissue may present an identical appearance. Glioma tissue may appear of slightly higher attenuation value than brain tissue without histological evidence of calcification or haemorrhage, but if significantly higher than brain attenuation, then these possibilities should be considered. Gliomas may grow predominantly by infiltration or by expansion and the CT appearance may reflect this. They may cross the midline by infiltrating the corpus callosum (Fig. 7.6). They may expand a single lobe to such an extent that the tumour may appear to involve an adjacent lobe or to have crossed the midline. Gliomas can, however, extend across fissures and involve adjacent lobes.

Attempts to correlate grade of tumour with CT appearance are not wholly satisfactory, but, in general, high grade tumours tend to show marked variation in attenuation and enhancement characteristics while low grade tumours tend to be hypodense and show minimal or no enhancement. A low grade glioma may sometimes appear as a discrete area of calcification with little or no soft tissue component. Malignant tumours may be partly cystic or necrotic, and these areas will not show enhancement (except in those rare cases in which contrast medium is seen to enter the cystic part and form fluid levels.

On the other hand a tumour mass which shows a thick irregular enhancing margin with a low attenuation, non-enhancing component cannot necessarily be interpreted as cystic or necrotic as the lack of enhancement may merely reflect the facts that extravasated contrast medium has not diffused into that area and that this part of the tumour does not contain a pathological circulation.

2. Metastasis

There is no absolute way to distinguish solitary metastasis from glioma, although presence of calcification strongly favours the latter. Non-enhancing metastases are exceptional. Metastases are of variable attenuation on plain scan. Sometimes they appear as enhancing rings, and resemble abscesses but a thick irregular wall favours a tumour. Metastases tend to generate considerable oedema in relation to their size (Fig. 7.7). Some metastases, especially malignant melanoma, present with haemor-

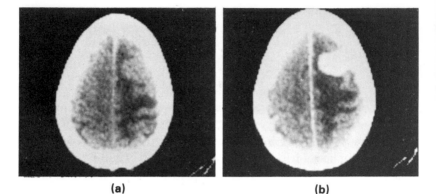

(a)   (b)

Fig. 7.7 (a, b)   Enhancing isodense metastasis with marked surrounding oedema.

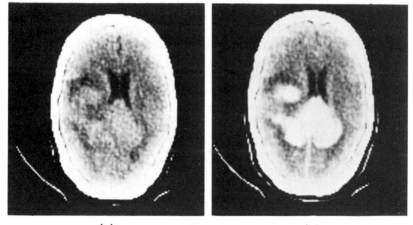
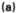

(a)   (b)

Fig. 7.8 (a, b)   Microglioma: slightly hyperdense, markedly enhancing masses, with peripheral oedema.

rhage and show blood attenuation on the plain scan. The diagnosis of metastatic disease is usually indicated by the presence of multiple lesions in a patient with a history of a known primary neoplasm.

Problems in diagnosis may be caused by multifocal neoplastic conditions such as microglioma and non-neoplastic conditions giving rise to multiple intracerebral lesions such as infarcts and granulomata.

3. Other Tumours

Lymphoma of the brain is more often primary (microglioma) than secondary. The CT features are those of intracerebral tumour, either solitary or multiple (Fig. 7.8). Although there is a spectrum of appearances, there is a tendency towards two distinct types of lesion on CT:

- (a) Infiltrating low attenuation, minimally or non-enhancing lesions, with a tendency to involve the periventricular tissues.
- (b) Discrete hyperdense and markedly enhancing masses with surrounding oedema.

Other malignant intracerebral tumours such as sarcoma, are rarities and specific diagnosis cannot be made from the CT scan.

4. Pineal Region Tumours

These lesions include true pineal cell tumours (pinealomas, of various degrees of malignancy), germinomas, teratomas and occasional gliomas and metastases. CT features are those of a tumour, indenting and compressing the posterior end of the third ventricle (Fig. 7.9). Anterior concavity of the posterior end of the third ventricle is an important sign as this differentiates a tumour from non-tumorous aqueduct stenosis. CT

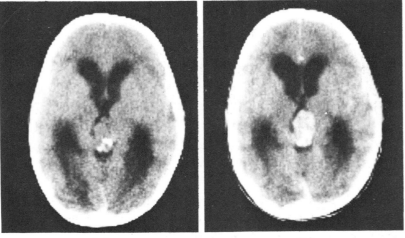

(a)   **(b)**

Fig. 7.9 (a, b) Pinealoma: irregular partially calcified mass indenting the back of the third ventricle and causing hydrocephalus with periventricular lucency. The quadrigeminal cistern is outlining the back of the tumour. Before and after contrast.

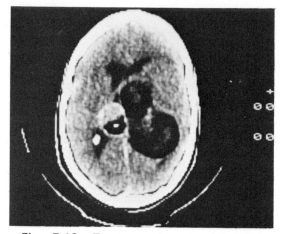

Fig. 7.10 Teratoma: Irregular lobulated mass containing tissues of fat and calcium density.

demonstrates the extent of the mass and the degree of associated hydrocephalus. Pinealomas and teratomas are more likely to be calcified than gliomas or metastases. Pinealomas usually show marked enhancement and tend to be round or lobulated masses, not infrequently with a cystic component. Glial tumours tend to show little or no enhancement. A teratoma is often very distinctive as it may contain calcium and fat (Fig. 7.10).

Pinealomas may extend into the midbrain, thalamic and hypothalamic regions, and occasionally arise more anteriorly in the third ventricle, in which case they may present with diabetes insipidus or precocious puberty. Some pathologists believe that these 'ectopic pinealomas' are, however, germinomas.

INFLAMMATORY LESIONS

1. Meningitis

This condition is included here only to stress that CT scan abnormalities are very rarely seen in uncomplicated pyogenic meningitis. The ventricles may be slightly dilated.

2. Pyogenic Abscess

CT is the radiological method of choice for diagnosis, localization and follow-up of intracranial abscesses. CT can detect the presence of two adjacent but discrete lesions which would appear as one confluent swelling at angiography, and similarly, can show the presence of multiple loculi in an abscess. CT will also show lesions smaller than may be detected by other radiological techniques. The plain scan finding is of an irregular area of low attenuation with mass effect. Frequently a slightly denser rim is visible within this region, which after contrast enhancement proves to be the wall of the abscess (Fig. 7.11). The enhancing ring is usually roughly spherical smooth and uniformly thin, and the contents of less than brain attenuation. Peripheral oedema is virtually always present, and this may be extensive. Absence of oedema is very unusual and should raise doubts about the diagnosis of abscess. The lesion may be multiloculated in which case the wall of each cavity may be distorted from the more typical spherical shape. Abscesses are usually of typical ring configuration by the time of CT diagnosis, but occasionally such lesions will be detected at the stage of 'cerebritis', i.e. before central necrosis has occurred, and the scan may demonstrate homogeneous enhancement. Diagnosis is difficult at this stage and a follow up scan should be performed.

3. Tuberculosis

Intracerebral tuberculous granulomata may mimic pyogenic abscesses if they have undergone sufficient central caseation (Fig. 7.12), although their centres are not usually as hypodense as those of pyogenic abscesses.

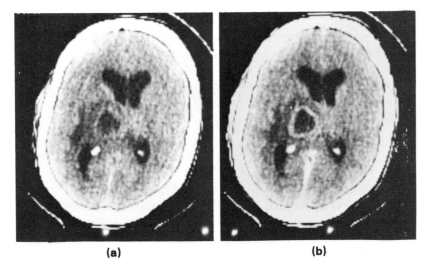

(a)   **(b)**

Fig. 7.11 (a, b)   Left thalamic abscess showing typical ring enhancement. Before and after contrast.

Granulomata, however, frequently show more mural irregularity or appear as solid enhancing lesions (Fig. 7.13a). There may be evidence of subarachnoid granulation tissues as evidenced by marked basal meningeal enhancement (Fig. 7.13b). A clue to this on the plain scan, is failure to visualise the basal cisterns. CT may in addition, demonstrate a complication such as hydrocephalus.

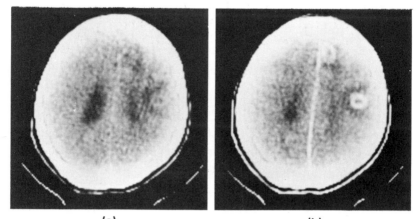

(a)   **(b)**

Fig. 7.12 (a, b) Enhancing rings with oedema. Tuberculous abscesses.

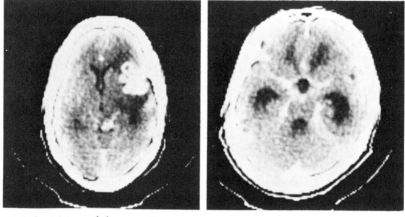

(a)   **(b)**

Fig. 7.13 (a) Enhanced scan showing tuberculous granuloma in right Sylvian region.
(b) Enhanced scan showing marked enhancement of basal meninges due to chronic granulomatous meningitis (tuberculosis).

4. Fungal Abscess

These lesions usually occur in patients on immunosuppressive therapy. They may show homogeneous or ring enhancement and are indistinguishable from pyogenic abscesses.

5. Encephalitis

In herpes simplex encephalitis CT frequently demonstrates low attenuation in the temporal lobe, frequently bilaterally. The low attenuation may, however, be more extensive and may be associated with swelling or areas of haemorrhage. Areas of contrast enhancement may be seen. Rapid and severe atrophic changes may be seen in the affected areas on follow up scans.

In other viral illnesses, non-specific areas of reduced white matter attenuation are occasionally seen, sometimes however only detectable in retrospect when comparison is made with follow up scans. Such conditions include measles, chicken-pox and Coxsackie virus infection.

6. Progressive Multifocal Leukoencephalopathy

This condition occurs in patients with an altered immune response and is due to a papovavirus infection. The CT findings are of somewhat irregular areas of reduced attenuation, predominantly in a white matter distribution but which may extend into grey matter. There may be associated mass effect, and there may be contrast enhancement, although this is not the rule. The CT abnormalities are usually multifocal, but a single area of affection may be encountered.

VASCULAR CONDITIONS

CT is of great value in strokes. An abnormality is shown more frequently than by conventional radiology; it permits the distinction between primary intracerebral haemorrhage and infarction, and localizes the lesion accurately. CT may also show an underlying tumour or arteriovenous malformation.

1. Intracerebral Haemorrhage

Spontaneous haemorrhage is shown as a relatively well-defined area of high attenuation (55–90 HU) (Fig. 7.14). A very early scan may show no peripheral low attenuation, but clot retraction and serum extrusion occur within hours and a thin rim of low attenuation is usually seen and is at least partly explained by this. There is often some oedema in the adjacent brain

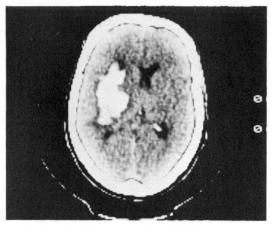

Fig. 7.14   Unenhanced scan: Spontaneous intracerebral haemorrhage with thin rim of surrounding low attenuation.

in addition, but less than that seen in cases of traumatic intracerebral haematoma. CT may demonstrate additional features such as intraventricular or subarachnoid extension of blood. The margins of the lesion often show ring enhancement with intravenous contrast after a few days and the high attenuation of the haematoma slowly decreases with time so that the lesion may become of low attenuation within one or two weeks. The haematoma is then slowly absorbed, frequently leaving a low attenuation area which may be indistinguishable from an infarct. An underlying cause for the haemorrhage is occasionally apparent (e.g. malignant tumour, angiomatous malformation or aneurysm) and contrast enhancement may help to make this diagnosis. It is not always easy to exclude an underlying lesion however, and in doubtful cases angiography is indicated.

2. Cerebral Infarction

The typical appearance of an infarct is that of a clearly defined area of low attenuation, in the distribution of a vascular territory (Fig. 7.15) Infarcts vary in size from small lacunar lesions (Fig. 7.16) to massive lesions involving an entire hemisphere. They are often multiple.

The appearance of an infarct and its pattern of enhancement change with time following the event:

(a) In the first few days the scan may be normal although more typically it shows low attenuation. Enhancement may occur as soon

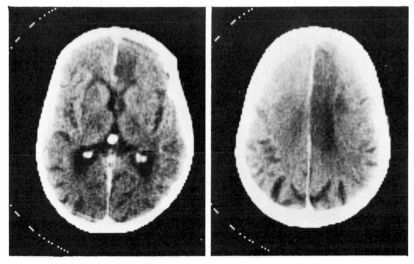

(a)　　　　　　　　(b)

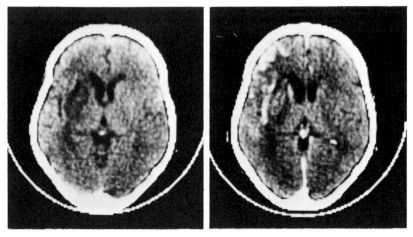

(c)　　　　　　　　(d)

Fig. 7.15 (a, b) Paramedian strip of low attenuation corresponding to anterior cerebral artery distribution. Right anterior cerebral infarct. **(c, d)** Reduced attenuation in left middle cerebral artery territory. After contrast: enhancement in the fronto-temporal cortex and deep structures (cortical and perforating vessel territories). Middle cerebral artery infarct.

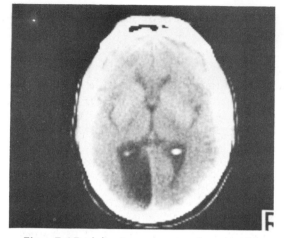

Fig. 7.15 (e) Low attenuation in left occipital lobe with dilatation of the adjacent ventricle. Mature left posterior cerebral infarct.

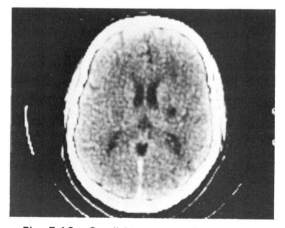

Fig. 7.16 Small low attenuation lesion in right lentiform region. Lacunar infarct.

as 6 hours after the event and may be seen in patients whose plain scan was normal. There may be evidence of mass effect, due to swelling of the ischaemic tissues.

(b) In the second and third weeks most infarcts that are large enough show a low attenuation area, and by the third week about 80% of infarcts show pathological enhancement (Fig. 7.17). Scans which previously showed low attenuation may transiently become isodense in the second week. This is thought to be due to exudation of blood from capillaries. Any mass effect, is usually maximal at this stage.

(c) After a month the proportion of infarcts which continue to enhance decreases progressively. Enhancement may now be peripheral due to ingrowth of capillaries. The apparent extent of the infarct tends to decrease and there is often accompanying local atrophy of the brain. This feature therefore suggests a mature infarct.

(d) Very few infarcts enhance after 3 months.

It is important to appreciate that the plain scan may appear normal in the presence of infarction in the following situations:

(a) First few days and second week
(b) Small lacunar infarcts (beyond resolution of scanner)
(c) Brain stem or posterior fossa infarcts (difficult areas to demonstrate clearly)
(d) Mildly haemorrhagic infarcts (isodense)

A haemorrhagic infarct (Fig. 7.18) may contain only small areas of haemorrhage which may render it isodense with adjacent brain. However, patchy areas of increased attenuation within a low attenuation region is the typical appearance. If the haemorrhagic element is marked, it may be difficult to distinguish from a primary haemorrhage. The term 'infarct' is

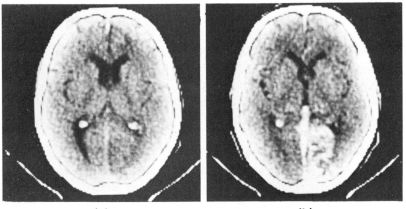

(a) **(b)**

Fig. 7.17 (a) Unenhanced scan — two weeks after sudden onset of right homonymous hemianopia, no low attenuation visible, but there is compression of the right occipital horn.
(b) Following contrast, marked enhancement in the right posterior cerebral distribution. Posterior cerebral infarct.

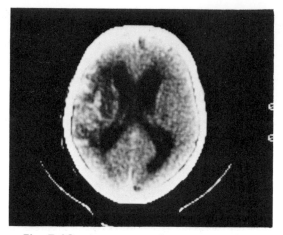

Fig. 7.18   Low attenuation area containing
areas of high (blood) attenuation in left middle
cerebral territory. Haemorrhagic infarct.

often used rather loosely to describe an area of low attenuation consequent
on vascular occlusion. Such an area of low attenuation may however
represent ischaemia rather than irreversible damage, especially in the
context of arterial spasm, and both the scan abnormality and clinical
deficit may resolve.

A watershed infarct (Fig. 7.19) is an area of infarction affecting the
tissues in the zone between two vascular territories and is typically due to
severe hypotension, for example following cardiac arrest.

When considering the possibility of cerebral infarction it must be
remembered that the scan may be normal in the early stages. Differential
diagnosis includes a tumour if the infarct has mass effect and occasionally
small lacunar lesions may be mistaken for plaques of multiple sclerosis.
The variable enhancement pattern may give rise to confusion with an
AVM.

There is at least a theoretical risk that iodinated contrast medium may
be toxic to neural tissue, especially if already damaged by ischaemia, and
contrast enhancement should not be carried out as a routine procedure in
cases of cerebral infarction, but be restricted to those cases in which it may
contribute positively.

3. Venous Occlusion

Although a normal scan is compatible with the diagnosis of obstruction
of the cortical veins or sinuses, the typical features are those of low attenu-

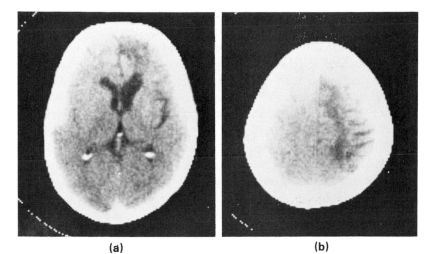

(a)   (b)

Fig. 7.19 (a, b)   Irregular low attenuation area between the anterior and middle cerebral artery territories. The lateral ventricle, Sylvian fissure and cortical sulci are enlarged on the right. Mature watershed infarct due to carotid occlusion.

ation, with swelling, involving one or both hemispheres particularly affecting the white matter, and occasionally containing focal areas of haemorrhage. Focal enhancement may be seen in these ischaemic areas.

Other Vascular Lesions

Hypertension and polycythaemia have been recorded as showing reduced attenuation in the cerebral white matter.

In malignant hypertension there may be ventricular compression due to diffuse swelling and possibly haemorrhage, occasionally multifocal. Chronic hypertension can be associated with low attenuation in a symmetrical periventricular distribution, predominantly in the frontal and parietal white matter, frequently extending into the anterior capsular regions. Atrophy is usually present in these cases and there is a high incidence of dementia in the clinical presentation.

A clotting defect may be suggested by multiple haemorrhages, which may be of lower attenuation than usual. Similar features may be seen in patients on anticoagulant therapy.

DEGENERATIVE CONDITIONS

Focal atrophy is the end result of many pathological processes. The loss of cerebral substance is usually indicated by widening of the adjacent CSF spaces, ventricular or subarachnoid. In neuronal degeneration, the main purpose of CT is to exclude underlying lesions such as tumour, or hydrocephalus in atypical cases. Non-specific atrophic change is the most frequent finding but more specific changes have been described including basal ganglia cavitation in some cases of Parkinsonism and Wilson's Disease and frontal horn enlargement due to caudate atrophy in Huntington's chorea.

Diffuse cerebral atrophy is diagnosed when the ventricles and subarachnoid spaces are shown to be enlarged. The degrees of enlargement should be approximately equal; ventricular dilatation in the presence of small or invisible sulci suggests hydrocephalus. Correlation of the degree of cerebral atrophy with dementia is poor, but ventricular enlargement correlates better than sulcal widening. Evan's Ratio was described as an aid to the assessment of ventricular enlargement: the ratio of the maximum dimension across the frontal horns to the maximum transverse internal skull diameter should not exceed 0·3 in the normal. However there is no doubt that ventricular dilatation may be present elsewhere in the system despite a normal Evan's Ratio. A list of the causes of atrophy is given in Chapter 8.

TOXIC AND METABOLIC LESIONS

Hepatic and renal failure have been reported to cause reduced attenuation in the cerebral hemispheres, predominantly in white matter.

Basal ganglia calcification is only very rarely associated with a metabolic disorder such as hyperparathyroidism and pseudohypoparathyroidism. It is seen so frequently that it may be considered a normal finding (Fig. 7.20).

Disseminated necrotizing leukoencephalopathy causes diffuse reduction in white matter attenuation in both hemispheres, associated with swelling, sometimes marked. Areas of calcification may be seen in the white matter and basal ganglia. The patients have usually been subjected to combined radiation and antimetabolite therapy, the latter most often being methotrexate. It is probable that the lesion represents brain damage caused by the antimetabolites which have crossed the blood-brain barrier following damage by radiation.

Carbon monoxide poisoning resulting in anoxic brain damage, may show basal ganglia cavitation, and diffuse atrophic change.

Chronic alcohol abuse is frequently associated with cerebral atrophy.

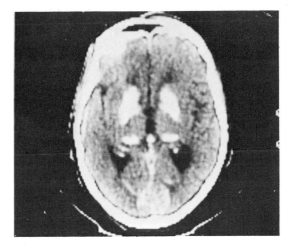

Fig. 7.20 Unusually extensive idiopathic calcification in the basal ganglia.

PARASITIC LESIONS

Hyatid cysts are seen as clear cut, spherical masses of CSF attenuation. They do not calcify. They show no enhancement except occasionally within adjacent compressed brain.

Cases of cysticercosis usually show sub-ependymal and intracerebral nodules which may be calcified. There may be hydrocephalus caused by an associated ependymitis. If the cysts die they may produce an intense inflammatory reaction in the cerebral substance.

MULTIPLE SCLEROSIS

Some cases of multiple sclerosis have the specific, if not pathognomonic CT appearance of relatively well-defined areas of low attenuation in the periventricular tissues, probably most frequently seen in the regions of the lateral ventricular trigones, and representing plaques of demyelination (Fig. 7.21). The lack of any mass effect is an important feature. Chronic plaques do not enhance but actively demyelinating areas may show enhancement (Fig. 7.22). Plaques may occasionally be isodense and only detected when they show enhancement with iodinated contrast medium. The more advanced cases almost invariably show evidence of diffuse atrophy. Confluent enhancing plaques may occasionally be mistaken for a glioma.

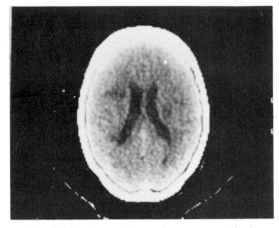

Fig. 7.21   Low attenuation paraventricular plaques in multiple sclerosis.

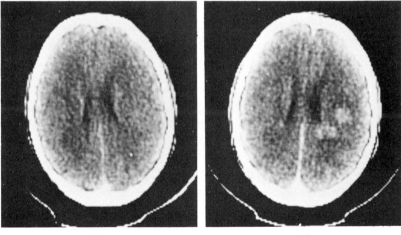

(a)   (b)

Fig. 7.22 (a, b)   Enhancing multiple sclerosis plaques not evident on the unenhanced scan. Before and after contrast.

Pathology	Tissue loss	Mass effect	Attenuation	Oedema	Enhancement
1. *Congenital* Leukodystrophy	As consequence of neuronal degeneration	–	Reduced in white matter	–	Occasionally (Adrenoleukodystrophy, Alexander's)
2. *Trauma* Contusion	Only as late sequela	+ (in acute stage)	Reduced or isodense; may contain high attenuation areas due to haemorrhage	+/–	–
Haematoma	End result may be a cavity	+	High with peripheral low attenuation	Often contributes to peripheral low attenuation	Sometimes peripheral enhancement around resolving haemorrhage
3. *Neoplasm* Glioma	–	+	Wide spectrum: low, high or mixed. May be calcified or contain blood	Usually	Frequently present, variable pattern, sometimes none

Pathology	Tissue loss	Mass effect	Attenuation	Oedema	Enhancement
Microglioma	–	+ (May be multiple)	Low attenuation infiltrating lesions, or hyperdense masses	Usually	Hyperdense masses usually enhance markedly
Metastasis	–	+ (May be multiple)	Low, high or mixed	+ (Often marked)	Almost invariably
4. *Inflammatory* Acute bacterial meningitis	–	–	Normal	–	–
Pyogenic abscess	–	+	Low attenuation; may contain discernible rim	+ (Often marked)	Ring
Granuloma	–	+	Usually slightly hyperdense	+	Homogeneous or ring; may have associated meningeal enhancement
Progressive multifocal leukoencephalopathy	–	Occasional slight. (May be single, or multiple)	Reduced in white matter (may extend into grey matter)	Probably contributes to reduced attenuation	Occasional

Pathology	Tissue loss	Mass effect	Attenuation	Oedema	Enhancement
Encephalitis	Sometimes marked atrophy in late stages	+ (May be marked)	Reduced, usually in white matter distribution	+	Occasional, e.g. herpes
5. *Vascular* Malignant hypertension	–	Sometimes swelling	Sometimes reduced in white matter; occasional haemorrhage	May contribute to reduced attenuation	–
Infarct	In later stages (mature infarct)	In acute stage; may be marked	Low unless haemorrhagic. Normal at some stages	Contributes to low attenuation	Frequently + in first month

Pathology	Tissue loss	Mass effect	Attenuation	Oedema	Enhancement
Haemorrhagic infarct	+ (In later stages)	+ (In acute stage)	Areas of high attenuation within low attenuation region	Contributory factor	Frequently + in first month
Venous occlusion	–	+ (May be marked)	Often normal, may be reduced, sometimes focal haemorrhage. White matter particularly affected	Contributory factor	Sometimes patchy enhancement
6. Metabolic Uraemia and hepatic failure	–	Sometimes swelling	Reduced in white matter	Probably contributes to reduced attenuation	–

CHAPTER EIGHT

The Ventricular System

CHANGES IN CONFIGURATION

(a) Enlargement
(b) Generalized compression
(c) Deformity

CHANGES IN ATTENUATION

(a) Diffuse or multifocal
(b) Focal

CHANGES IN CONFIGURATION AND ATTENUATION

Intraventricular tumours

1. CHANGES IN CONFIGURATION

(a) Enlargement
(i) *Generalized*

	Pathology	Comment
Lateral, third and fourth ventricles:	Atrophy (combined cerebral and cerebellar)	
	Communicating hydrocephalus	
	Obstructive hydro-cephalus	− Fourth ventricle outlet foramina

1. CHANGES IN CONFIGURATION
(*continued*)

(a) Enlargement
(i) *Generalized*

	Pathology	Comment
Lateral and third ventricles:	Cerebral atrophy Communicating hydrocephalus	– Fourth ventricle is frequently normal in size
	Obstructive hydrocephalus	– Posterior end of third ventricle (pinealoma) – Aqueduct – Posterior fossa masses
Both lateral ventricles:	Cerebral atrophy Obstructive hydrocephalus	– Both interventricular foramina – Third ventricle
	Communicating hydrocephalus	

(ii) *Focal*

	Pathology	Site
One lateral ventricle:	Hydrocephalus	Obstruction of interventricular foramen
	Hemi-atrophy	
Part of a lateral ventricle:	Focal atrophy Focal obstructive hydrocephalus	– loculated ventricle

A frequent problem in differential diagnosis is that between atrophy and hydrocephalus. The ventricular enlargement in cerebral atrophy is in proportion to the widening of the subarachnoid spaces (Fig. 8.1) whereas in hydrocephalus due to an obstruction in the ventricular pathways the ventricular dilatation is the striking feature, the sulci being small or effaced. Visualization of an obstructing lesion with dilatation of the ventricles above the block often makes the diagnosis simple. Even without demonstration of a mass lesion, the discrepancy in the ventricular dilatation may indicate the level of obstruction, as for example in benign

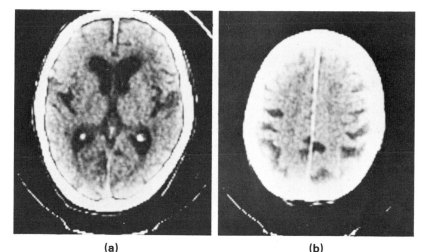

(a)   **(b)**

Fig. 8.1 (a, b)   Enlarged ventricles and subarachnoid spaces. Cerebral atrophy.

aqueduct stenosis, where third and lateral ventricular dilatation is seen in the presence of a small or normal sized fourth ventricle.

In communicating hydrocephalus all the ventricles may be enlarged, but frequently the third and fourth ventricles are not strikingly so.

The subarachnoid spaces may also be dilated, depending on the underlying cause, so that basal cisterns, Sylvian fissures and parts of the interhemispheric fissure may be enlarged in the presence of a high convexity absorption block, making the differential diagnosis from atrophy very difficult, sometimes impossible. There are probably many cases where the two conditions co-exist.

Reduced attenuation in the periventricular tissue, referred to as periventricular lucency (PVL) (Fig. 8.2) is seen in some cases of hydrocephalus, both obstructive and communicating. It is present most frequently in the frontal region, but also occurs in temporal, occipital and parietal regions (in reducing incidence). It has to be distinguished from white matter low attenuation which may be seen in many differing conditions and may cause difficulty in diagnosis when associated with enlarged ventricles in older patients with chronic vascular hypertension who in fact have ischaemic white matter changes and cerebral atrophy (Fig. 8.3).

A list of causes of the appearance of cerebral atrophy on CT scans is given on p. 88.

A list of the causes of hydrocephalus is given on p. 89.

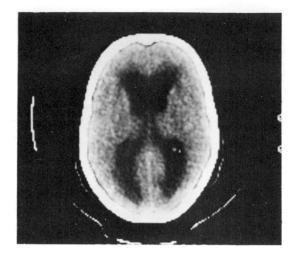

Fig. 8.2 Dilated lateral ventricles with periventricular lucency. Hydrocephalus.

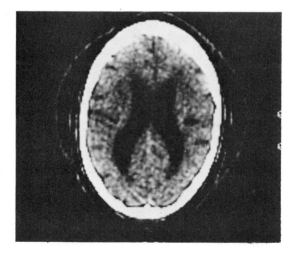

Fig. 8.3 Cerebral atrophy: enlarged lateral ventricles and cortical sulci, with low attenuation in the white matter adjacement to the bodies of the lateral ventricles.

1(b) Generalized Compression of the Lateral Ventricles

	Pathology	
One lateral ventricle	Extracerebral collection	
	Hemisphere swelling (post-op, traumatic)	
	Extensive infarct	
	Occasionally diffuse tumour	
Both lateral ventricles	Bilateral isodense extracerebral collections	
	Diffuse brain swelling	– trauma
		encephalitis
		sinus thrombosis
	(Benign intracranial hypertension)	

It may only become evident after follow-up scans that the ventricles were diffusely compressed in some conditions. There is no absolute lower limit of normal size for the ventricles; some normal scans show ventricles which are barely visible. However, in old age the lateral ventricles usually show at least moderate dilatation, and demonstration of very small ventricles in this age group is suggestive of compression.

1(c) Deformity of Ventricles

	Pathology	
Lateral ventricle	Hemisphere mass lesion	– tumour
		– infarct
		haemorrhage
		– extracerebral
		mass lesion
Common lateral ventricle	Absent septum	
Third ventricle	Pinealoma posteriorly	
	Deep tumour, haemorrhage, infarct	
Fourth ventricle	Brainstem cerebellar or fourth ventricular mass	
	Extrinsic mass	

Focal deformity of a ventricle indicates a relatively deep focal lesion in proximity to the ventricle whereas compression of an entire lateral ventricle suggests a more diffuse lesion, which may be in the hemisphere or extracerebral.

A CSF attenuation midline cleft between the frontal horns characterizes a cavum septi pellucidi which is a normal variant. A more extensive anomaly is seen when a posterior extension of this cleft is present between the bodies of the lateral ventricles (cavum vergae).

2. CHANGES IN ATTENUATION

(a) diffuse

increase   – intraventricular haemorrhage (Fig. 8.4)
contrast medium (Metrizamide)
intraventricular spread of tumour

(b) focal or multifocal

(i) increase   – blood
– myodil
– calcification – choroid plexus
– paraventricular masses in tuberose sclerosis
– periventricular calcification in toxoplasmosis
– primary intraventricular mass
colloid cyst of 3rd ventricle
meningioma
choroid plexus papilloma
– tumour invading ventricle
glioma
pinealoma
microglioma

(ii) decrease   – air – trauma
post-operative, lumbar puncture/AEG
fat – ruptured intracranial dermoid/epidermoid

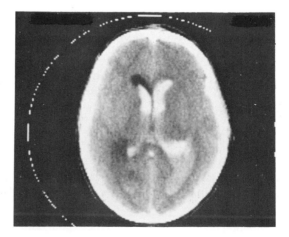

Fig. 8.4   Diffuse intraventricular haemorrhage.

3. ABNORMAL ATTENUATION AND CONFIGURATION

	Intraventricular masses	*Primary extraventricular masses apparently intraventricular*
Lateral ventricles	Meningioma (Fig. 8.5) Choroid plexus papilloma Microglioma	Ependymoma Glioma (Fig. 8.6) Metastasis Arteriovenous malformation (Fig. 8.7) Haemorrhage
Third ventricle	Colloid cyst (Fig. 8.8) Metastases from pineal region tumour	Pinealoma Glioma Craniopharyngioma Basilar artery ectasia/ aneurysm
Fourth ventricle (see Chapter 11)		

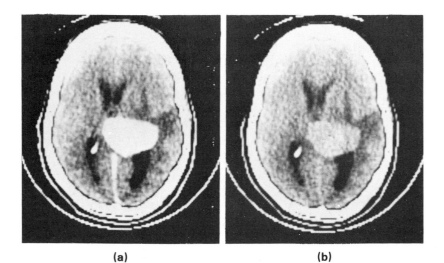

(a)   (b)

Fig. 8.5 (a, b) Hyperdense markedly enhancing mass centred on the left trigone. Intraventricular meningioma.

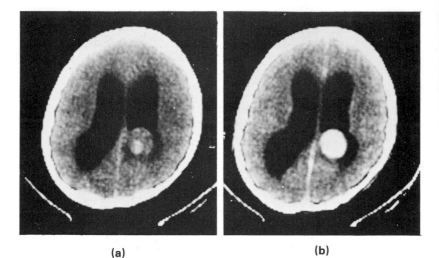

(a)   (b)

Fig. 8.6 (a, b)   Astrocytoma extending into the ventricle: before and after contrast enhancement.

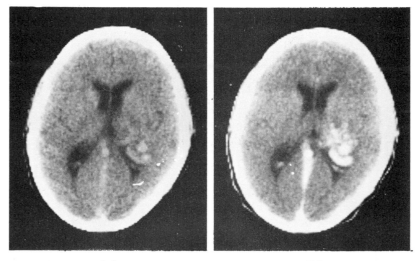

(a)   (b)

Fig. 8.7 (a, b)   Angiomatous malformation deforming right trigone: before and after contrast enhancement.
(c) (*opposite*)   Coronal scan showing intraventricular extent.

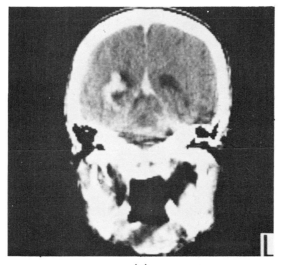

(c)

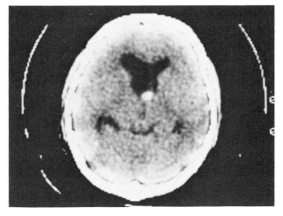

Fig. 8.8 Colloid cyst obstructing the left foramen of Munro.

It is frequently difficult to decide whether a tumour is situated inside or outside a ventricle. It is also difficult to decide whether a tumour which has arisen from an extraventricular site adjacent to a ventricle, is growing into and involving the ventricle or only appearing to do so by deforming the ventricular wall.

Colloid cyst: this is seen as a small round hyperdense mass in the anterior third ventricle in the region of the foramen of Munro. It does not usually enhance visibly with contrast. There is often associated hydrocephalus of one or both lateral ventricles.

Choroid plexus papilloma: a hyperdense mass most frequently arising in the region of the trigone of the lateral ventricle which enhances markedly with contrast. It may simulate an intraventricular meningiona.

CAUSES OF 'RADIOLOGICAL ATROPHY'

1. Generalized:
    Senile involution
    Alzheimer's disease
    Chronic alcohol abuse
    Anoxia
    Radiotherapy
    System degenerations
    Huntington's chorea
    Hydrocephalus (apparent after shunting)
    Head injury
    Multiple sclerosis
    Multiple infarcts
    Binswinger's disease
    Steroids (reversible sulcal enlargement)
    Dehydration (reversible)
    Connective tissue disorders, e.g. S.L.E., P.A.N.
    Post-viral encephalitis including herpes
    Jakob-Creutzfeld disease (rapidly progressive atrophy)
    Storage disorders (leukodystrophy and mucopolysaccharidoses)
    Marasmus
    Chronic epilepsy (disputed)

In some of the above conditions, generalized atrophy is not necessarily the only abnormality and parenchymal lesions may be seen in addition.

2. Focal:
Almost all conditions which can cause generalized atrophy may occur in an asymmetrical pattern, affecting one part of the brain more than others, but atrophy in the following conditions is characteristically focal.

Trauma	Radiotherapy
Old infarction	Post-herpes encephalitis
Old haemorrhage	Sturge-Weber syndrome
Surgery	

CAUSES OF HYDROCEPHALUS

(a) Communicating

   (i)   Subarachnoid haemorrhage

  (ii)   Sequela of meningitis

 (iii)   Granulomatous or neoplastic meningeal infiltration

(b) Obstructive

(i) Outlet of 4th ventricle	Congenital atresia
	Arnold-Chiari malformation
	Tumour
	Post infective
(ii) At the level of 4th ventricle	Tumour involving 4th ventricle (intraventricular, brainstem, cerebellar, extrinsic)
(iii) At aqueduct level	Benign aqueduct stenosis
	Neoplastic stenosis
	Kinking
(iv) Third ventricle	Tumour – pineal region
	– thalamus
	– colloid cyst
	– craniopharyngioma
	– pituitary tumour
(v) At Foramina of Munro	Colloid cyst
	Glioma
	Compression due to hemisphere mass
(vi) Part of the lateral ventricle	Intraventricular tumour (q.v.)
	Tumour compressing ventricle
	Post inflammatory ependymitis

Synopsis to Chapter Nine

1. SUBARACHNOID SPACE

(a) Changes in configuration

  (i) Dilatation
  (ii) Diminution
  (iii) Non-visualization

(b) Change from CSF attenuation

  (i) Greater than brain attenuation
  (ii) Equal to brain attenuation
  (iii) Less than CSF attenuation

2. EXTRACEREBRAL MASS LESIONS

(a) Greater than brain attenuation
(b) Isodense
(c) Less than brain attenuation

The Extracerebral Space

1. SUBARACHNOID SPACE

(a) Changes in configuration
(i) Dilatation
Diffuse widening
Atrophy – cerebrum, cerebellum, brainstem
Focal widening
Focal atrophy
Communicating hydrocephalus – below absorption block

Extrinsic mass	– widens space by displacing neuraxis, e.g. acoustic neuroma displacing brainstem and therefore widening cisterns adjacent to tumour
Intrinsic mass	– exophytic extension may cause same effect as extrinsic mass

Arachnoid cyst (Fig. 9.1)
Epidermoid

(ii) Diminution
Diffuse reduction
Diffuse brain swelling
Hydrocephalus
Extracerebral collection (Fig. 9.2)
Focal reduction
Intrinsic mass
Extrinsic mass
Transtentorial coning – e.g. temporal lobe encroaching on chiasmatic cistern, brainstem encroaching on pontine cistern

(iii) Non-visualization

Mass effect	— Cerebral swelling
	— hydrocephalus
	— extracerebral collection
	— meningeal infiltration (tumour or granuloma)
Isodense CSF	— subarachnoid haemorrhage (6–10 days after haemorrhage)

(b) Change from CSF attenuation

(i) Greater than brain attenuation

Diffuse

Subarachnoid haemorrhage (Fig. 9.3) — first few days following haemorrhage

Focal

Subarachnoid blood

Calcification — vascular
— TB meningitis

Myodil

Aneurysm, ectasia

(ii) Equal to brain attenuation

Subarachnoid haemorrhage — 6–10 days old

Meningeal infiltration — granulomatous, neoplastic

(iii) Less than CSF attenuation

Fat — lipoma
— ruptured dermoid
— epidermoid

Air — post-operative (or AEG) post-traumatic post lumbar puncture

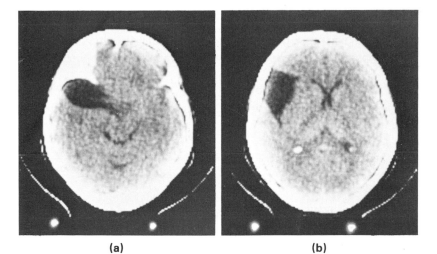

(a)   (b)

Fig. 9.1 (a, b) Left sylvian region arachnoid cyst extending to chiasmatic cistern. There is left temporal lobe hypoplasia and only slight mass effect.

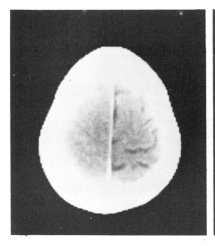

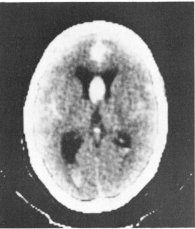

Fig. 9.2 Effacement of cortical sulci by left subdural collection.

Fig. 9.3 Haemorrhage from anterior communicating artery aneurysm. Blood is seen in the septum pellucidum, the occipital horns as well as in the inter-hemispheric and both sylvian fissures.

2. EXTRACEREBRAL MASS LESIONS

Extra-axial masses restricted to specific anatomical situations such as the CP angle and the posterior fossa are listed under those headings.

(a) Greater than brain attenuation

Acute subdural haematoma	– high attenuation for first 10 days
Extradural haematoma	
Meningioma	
Chordoma	

(b) Isodense

Subdural haematoma	– isodense phase 10–20 days
Meningioma	– occasionally isodense

(c) Less than brain attenuation

Chronic subdural haematoma	– more than 14 days old
Occasional meningioma	– enhances
Arachnoid cyst	– often middle fossa with temporal lobe hypoplasia
Epidermoid	

Lymphoma and metastatic disease may be found in the extracerebral spaces, and show a variable attenuation and enhancement pattern.

Meningioma: this is an extrinsic mass arising from the meninges of the skull base, vault, falx or tentorium (Fig. 9.4). Rarely (2%) it arises in a ventricle from the tela choroidea. The tumour is typically well circumscribed and grows by expansion, burrowing into adjacent brain. It may thus simulate an intracerebral tumour. There may be visible thickening of the bone at the site of attachment to the dura. The attenuation is typically greater than brain and it may contain calcification, although it may be isodense or even of low attenuation (Fig. 9.5). Sometimes cystic elements may be seen. Meningiomas may be associated with very extensive oedema although occasionally there is little or none. Enhancement is typically dense and fairly homogeneous, this being a characteristic diagnostic feature.

Extradural and subdural haematoma: extradural and subdural haematomas are frequently associated with trauma. They are both readily seen on a scan as high attenuation if the scan is taken within about seven days: after this time the blood becomes isodense with brain tissue. A

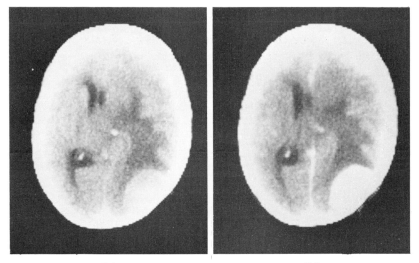

(a) (b)

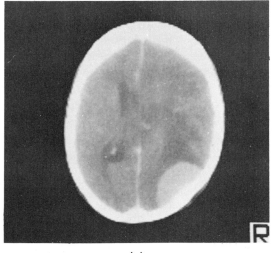

(c)

Fig. 9.4 (a, b) Convexity meningioma: raised attenuation mass showing marked enhancement. Extensive oedema. Before and after contrast.
(c) Image taken with a window width of 100 reveals hyperostosis at the site of attachment.

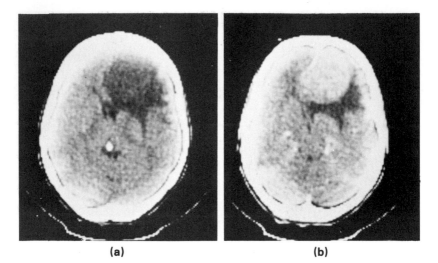

(a)   (b)

Fig. 9.5 (a, b)   Low attenuation meningioma: before and after contrast enhancement.

typical extradural haematoma is convex inwards (Fig. 9.6) and may be associated with a fracture. A subdural haematoma is less localized, tending to spread diffusely through the subdural space, its internal margin roughly paralleling the vault, being concave inwards. It may be difficult to detect mass effect if the lesions are bilateral. An isodense subdural haematoma is only revealed by the presence of mass effect and the non-visualization of cortical sulci on the side of the lesion. Diagnosis of an isodense subdural is only rarely aided by contrast enhancement when either the cortical vessels of the underlying brain, or the capsule will occasionally delineate it. Bilateral symmetrical isodense subdural haematomas are uncommon, but in such cases the lateral ventricles may appear small in relation to the patient's age suggesting bilateral compression. Medial displacement of the frontal horns is a helpful sign in suggesting such compression.

A subdural haematoma becomes hypodense after about 2–3 weeks and often develops a fairly thick capsule (Fig. 9.7). When such a capsule enhances markedly, the possibility of an infected subdural effusion is raised, but such enhancement can certainly occur in the absence of any infection.

Subarachnoid haemorrhage: subarachnoid haemorrhage can be diagnosed with great accuracy in the first few days immediately following the event, when the extravasated blood is seen as high attenuation replac-

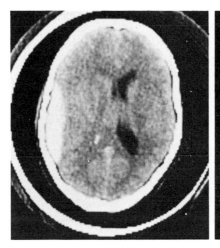
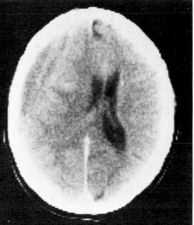

Fig. 9.6 Acute extradural haematoma; left hemisphere swelling adds to the mass effect.

Fig. 9.7 Low attenuation subdural collection.

ing the CSF attenuation of the subarachnoid spaces, most obvious in the basal cisterns but also detectable over the convexity and often associated with local intrusion of blood into the brain close to the site of the haemorrhage. After this time, there is a period in which the blood-CSF mixture in the cisterns is isodense with brain, resulting in failure to visualize the CSF spaces. Ten days or so after haemorrhage, the CSF spaces have usually reverted to normal CSF attenuation. The distribution of the subarachnoid blood sometimes indicates the likely site of aneurysm, and may be helpful in planning angiography. Hydrocephalus may develop within a very short period following subarachnoid haemorrhage and be evident at the time of initial scan. About 10% of scans may be normal even in the first week.

CHAPTER TEN

Lesions of the Sella and Juxtasellar Region

This region is the site of a variety of lesions, and careful study of the CT features frequently allows specific diagnosis. In the following discussion the lesions are classified according to their site; use of this system in differential diagnosis will ensure that all important diagnostic possibilities are considered, even though in many cases the actual site of origin may not be precisely determinable. Further detail of a suprasellar mass may be shown on coronal cuts. A fairly recent development is CT following metrizamide enhancement of the CSF spaces, when cuts demonstrate any suprasellar mass as a filling defect within the opacified chiasmatic cistern. This technique may be especially valuable when axial and coronal scans are made, so building up a detailed three-dimensional anatomical display.

LESIONS WITHIN THE SELLA

Pituitary adenoma	– enlarged sella
	– variable attenuation and enhancement
Craniopharyngioma	– only 5% purely intrasellar
	– calcification strongly suggestive
Empty sella	– CSF attenuation

LESIONS IN SUPRASELLAR REGION

Pituitary adenoma	– continuity with intrasellar expanding mass
Craniopharyngioma	– frequent calcification
Meningioma	– usually typical attenuation, occasional hyperostosis detectable
Aneurysm	
Optic chiasm glioma	
Arachnoid cyst	– CSF attenuation
Epidermoid	– low attenuation

LESIONS IN LATERAL JUXTASELLAR REGION

Pituitary adenoma	– large tumours may extend into cavernous and medial temporal regions
Carotid aneurysm	– typical enhancement pattern
Meningioma	– cavernous region
Glioma	– temporal lobe
Hamartoma	

LESIONS IN POSTERIOR JUXTASELLAR REGION

Pituitary adenoma	– often extends into interpeduncular fossa
Craniopharyngioma	– retroclival extension not infrequent
Basilar aneurysm/ectasia	– nodular or fusiform enhancement
Chordoma	– commonly arises in clivus region
	– bone destruction, calcification

LESIONS ARISING FROM SKULL BASE

Chordoma	– bone destruction
	– calcified mass
Clivus meningioma	– typical enhancement
Sinus lesions	

LESIONS WITHIN THE SELLA

Pituitary tumour.   Pituitary tumour is the most common lesion in this area, and all other masses in the sellar region have to be differentiated from it. A pituitary tumour is typically homogeneous and hyperdense and usually enhances quite markedly (Fig. 10.1). The tumour usually expands the sella and frequently extends superiorly into the chiasmatic cistern towards the third ventricle, posteriorly into the interpeduncular fossa, laterally towards the temporal lobe and rather less frequently anteriorly into the inferior frontal region. Pituitary adenoma is sometimes of low attenuation, and cystic components, which may sometimes be large, are quite common.

Empty sella.   An extension of the subarachnoid space through the diaphragma sellae into the pituitary fossa is referred to as an empty sella, although usually there is a rim of pituitary tissue within the fossa. The sella is usually slightly expanded but this may be difficult to demonstrate by CT.

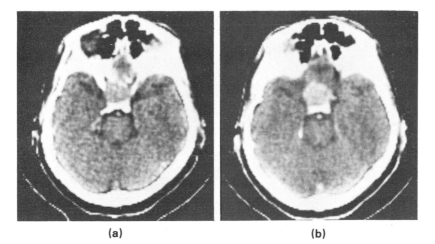

(a)   (b)

Fig. 10.1 (a, b) Hyperdense enhancing pituitary tumour in an expanded sella. Before and after contrast.

Caution must be observed in making this diagnosis, particularly if thick (10 or 13 mm) slices are used, because the partial volume effect of sphenoid sinus air or chiasmatic cistern CSF may lead to erroneous diagnosis. The condition of empty sella is frequently an incidental finding; on the other hand pituitary gland infarction may lead to it and it is occasionally seen in association with benign intracranial hypertension.

LESIONS IN SUPRASELLAR AND JUXTASELLAR REGIONS

Craniopharyngioma. This is a relatively common lesion, which is frequently associated with hydrocephalus. The lesions are usually of mixed attenuation, containing calcification in the majority of children and in 50% of adults; 5% are entirely intrasellar. The typical example contains solid and cystic components, and this is reflected in the CT image (Fig. 10.2), the solid portion enhancing, unlike the cystic low attenuation contents. There may be an enhancing capsule in relation to the cyst which may sometimes be simulated by vessels draped around the lesion. The mass may enlarge the sella from above but this is unusual. These lesions are almost always situated in the midline. Anterior extension is uncommon though posterior and retroclival extension is not infrequent. Hydrocephalus is frequently present with the larger masses.

Meningioma. Meningioma arising from the region of the planum

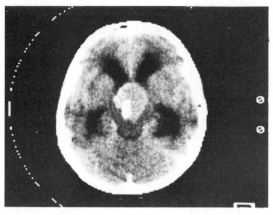

Fig. 10.2 Hyperdense partially calcified mass in the suprasellar region obliterating the third ventricle and causing hydrocephalus. Craniopharyngioma.

sphenoidale and tuberculum sellae presents as a suprasellar mass. Associated hyperostosis may be detectable by CT and will make specific diagnosis possible. The differential diagnosis in this region is usually between meningioma, suprasellar extension of pituitary tumour and suprasellar aneurysm. The meningioma is typically slightly hyperdense on plain scan, and shows marked but often not quite homogeneous enhancement (Fig. 10.3). There may be oedema in the adjacent brain tissue. The planum sphenoidale meningioma arises anterior to the sella but may extend posteriorly and is frequently attached also to the diaphragma sellae and then will present as a truly suprasellar mass.

Aneurysm.   An aneurysm encroaching on the suprasellar area may arise from any part of the circle of Willis or terminal carotid artery including the ophthalmic artery origin. The mass is slightly hyperdense on plain scan and may show marginal calcification (Fig. 10.4). The patent lumen shows marked homogeneous enhancement after contrast injection, but the enhancement pattern may be irregular due to the presence of mural thrombus, resulting in a peripheral non-enhancing component. This is generally the opposite pattern to inhomogeneous tumour enhancement and is a useful feature in differential diagnosis, but giant aneurysms occasionally show ring enhancement due to surrounding vascular adhesions. Coronal cuts may be very useful in demonstrating the suprasellar situation of aneurysms.

Arachnoid cyst.   The suprasellar region is one of the characteristic sites

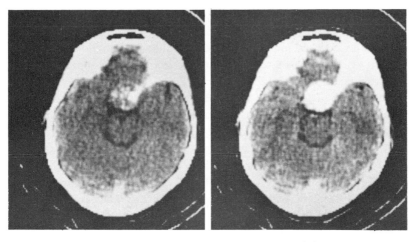

(a)   (b)

Fig. 10.3 (a) Hyperdense irregularly calcified meningioma arising from the tuberculum sellae. There is hyperostosis of the right sphenoid ridge medially.
(b) Marked enhancement after contrast.

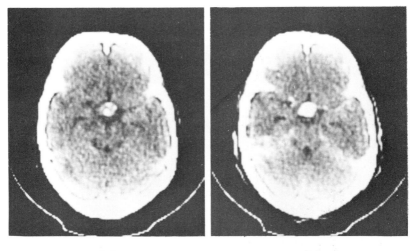

(a)   (b)

Fig. 10.4 (a, b) Small suprasellar mass showing marginal calcification. Marked enhancement after contrast. Anterior communicating artery aneurysm.

for this lesion which will be of CSF attenuation value on measurement (Fig. 10.5). It may obstruct the third ventricle causing hydrocephalus. Arachnoid cysts do not calcify or show enhancement. Not infrequently, there is evidence of extension of the cyst into the middle or posterior fossa subarachnoid spaces.

Epidermoid.   The distinction between epidermoid and arachnoid cyst is frequently difficult to make. Sometimes the lesion contains sufficient fatty tissue to suggest the diagnosis. An epidermoid may, however, be isodense and occasionally of raised attenuation. Marginal enhancement is sometimes present. These lesions tend to be situated laterally in the middle fossa but may extend up to the midline (Fig. 10.6). They extend into and enlarge CSF spaces, widening crural, ambient and other cisterns.

Optic chiasm glioma.   This lesion may represent the intracranial extension of an optic nerve glioma (seen as a fusiform optic nerve swelling and a widened optic canal on orbital views), or may arise primarily in the chiasm. It is seen most frequently in association with neurofibromatosis. It usually presents as a well defined mixed attenuation suprasellar mass, often with striking enhancement. Although it behaves as a benign tumour (?hamartomatous) it may invade locally to give a huge intracranial mass, burrowing into the brain usually following the path of the optic tracts frequently with cystic components. Calification occurs only after irradiation.

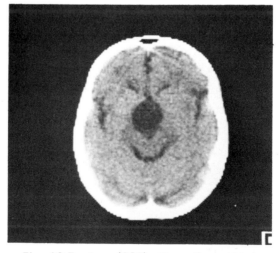

Fig. 10.5   Low (CSF) attenuation mass in chiasmatic cistern. Arachnoid cyst.

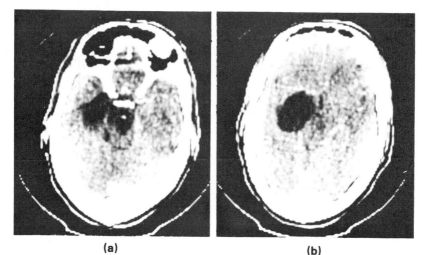

(a)   (b)

Fig. 10.6 (a, b) Low attenuation mass in the left medial temporal region extending behind the dorsum sellae into the posterior fossa. Epidermoid.

Hypothalamic gliomas. These tumours behave as more invasive and malignant masses, often with more irregular margins, than chiasm glioma, but are often difficult to differentiate from them.

Other suprasellar masses include relatively rare lesions such as germinoma of the anterior third ventricle and metastases.

LESIONS INVOLVING THE BASE AND ENCROACHING ON THE SELLAR REGION

Sinus Lesions

Expanding processes of the paranasal sinuses may encroach on the sellar region. Neoplasm and mucocele of the ethmoid or sphenoid sinus occasionally present in this way, as well as giant polyp which can occasionally present as a markedly expanding lesion. In benign conditions, the bony margins actually remain intact for a very long time although they may be markedly distorted and thinned, whereas bone destruction is a cardinal sign of malignant disease. Difficulties arise when very thin bone does not show up on the scan and looks as though it were eroded.

Nasopharyngeal Carcinoma

The tumour may erode the skull base and present in the juxtasellar region.

Chordoma

The mass usually arises within the clivus and erodes the sphenoid bone giving rise to a mass behind the clivus which compresses the brain stem. The tumour may extend into the nasopharynx. The typical CT features are of a partially calcified mass associated with bone destruction in the clivus region. A degree of enhancement may be seen in the tumour.

CHAPTER ELEVEN

The Posterior Fossa

The posterior fossa is the intracranial compartment below the tentorium cerebelli and contains the cerebellum, and most of the brainstem (midbrain, pons and medulla oblongata).

The boundaries of the posterior fossa are difficult to define on axial CT scans as the upper free edge of the tentorium through which the brainstem passes is at a higher level than the peripheral bony attachments. The lower limit of the posterior fossa is the skull base and foramen magnum. The anterolateral limits are the petrous ridges and the apex of the posterior fossa is approximately indicated by the pineal gland. The tentorial hiatus lies in the plane between the tip of the dorsum sellae and the pineal region. This complex configuration of the posterior fossa results in the upper midline portion of the posterior fossa being included in cuts which may also be demonstrating such supratentorial structures as the lateral ventricles. The tentorium is only occasionally visible on plain scan, but is very frequently visible on enhanced scans as a hazy zone of density with which the observer soon becomes familiar. Because the tent slopes upwards and medially, the tissues lateral to the tentorial margins are supratentorial, and those medial to the margins are infratentorial. Sometimes a pathological process may be present on both sides of the tentorium (e.g. meningioma), and coronal cuts may be very helpful in defining detailed anatomy.

LESIONS OF THE POSTERIOR FOSSA

1. Lesions within the subarachnoid space
2. Lesions involving the fourth ventricle
3. Lesions of the cerebellum
4. Lesions of the brainstem

1. Lesions within Subarachnoid Space

(i) Configuration change

(a) *Widening of subarachnoid spaces*

Large cisterna magna	– normal (wide variation in size)
CP angle cisterns	– unilateral widening by CP angle mass displacing neuraxis
	– bilateral widening in atrophy
Large superior cerebellar cistern	– normal (wide variation in size)
	– arachnoid cyst within it
All CSF spaces of posterior fossa (Fig. 11.1)	– cerebellar and brainstem atrophy
Widened cerebellar sulci	– cerebellar atrophy

(b) *Apparent diminution of subarachnoid spaces*

Diffuse	– normal variant (often technical)
	– isodense CSF – blood mixture after subarachnoid haemorrhage
Local	– encroachment by mass – intra-axial
	– extra-axial

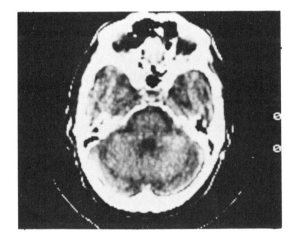

Fig. 11.1 Prominent fourth ventricle, cerebellar sulci and cisterns around the brainstem. Cerebellar and possible brainstem atrophy.

The size of the subarachnoid space is very variable. In particular the cisterna magna and superior cerebellar cisterns may be large in normality and their size is not a reliable criterion for the diagnosis of cerebellar atrophy; fourth ventricular and cerebellar sulcal enlargement in combination is the most reliable evidence.

An extra-axial mass in the subarachnoid space may be isodense and result in apparent diminution of the CSF space, but will often increase the size of the adjacent space by displacing the neuraxis. Similar effects may be caused by an exophytic extension from an intra-axial lesion.

(ii) Diffuse Attenuation Change

(a) *Increased attenuation of subarachnoid space*
Blood (recent subarachnoid haemorrhage)
Metrizamide

(b) *Reduced attenuation*   – fat or air

(iii) Mass lesion in subarachnoid space

(a) *Low attenuation*
Arachnoid cyst   – CSF attenuation
Epidermoid   – attenuation may be that of fat
                        – occasional marginal calcium
                        – occasional enhancement

(b) *Brain attenuation*
Acoustic neuroma
Meningioma (sometimes)

An acoustic neuroma always arises from the internal auditory meatus, although it may extend some distance, even into the middle fossa. The differential diagnosis from meningioma is only difficult when the meningioma arises at the same site. Acoustic neuroma is a much commoner lesion.

(c) *High attenuation*
Meningioma (Fig. 11.2)   – marked enhancement
Basilar artery aneurysm/   – enhancement of nodular or tubular
ectasia   structure
Chordoma   – usually visible bone destruction, calcium
                        – some enhancement
Epidermoid (rarely)

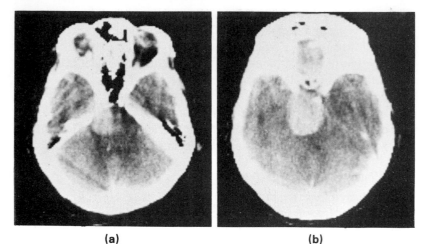

(a)   **(b)**

Fig. 11.2 (a, b)   Post contrast scans: petro-clival meningioma – large mass anterior to the brain stem.

(iv) **Cerebellopontine angle lesions** – lesions at this site are considered separately as they constitute a common and important differential diagnostic group.

	Typical attenuation	*Enhancement*
Acoustic neuroma (Fig. 11.3)	Isodense, occasional low attenuation cystic component	Usually marked
Meningioma	Hyperdense	Usually marked and homogeneous
Epidermoid	Hypodense	Occasional slight marginal enhancement
Glomus jugulare tumour	Isodense usually	Usually some, but difficult to demonstrate
Intrinsic lesion encroaching on CPA, e.g. exophytic glioma, metastasis	Variable	Variable
Ectatic basilar artery (Fig. 11.4)	Hyperdense ± calcium	Enhancement of patent lumen
Fifth nerve neuroma	Hyperdense	Usually marked

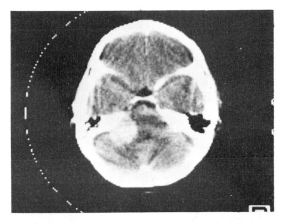

Fig. 11.3 Enhancing mass in the left cerebello-pontine angle, centred on the internal auditory meatus. Acoustic neuroma. (The mass was isodense prior to contrast injection.)

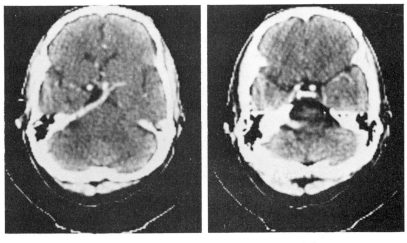

(a) (b)

Fig. 11.4 (a) Enhanced scan showing tortuous ectatic basilar artery. in a patient with trigeminal neuralgia.

(b) The lower continuation of the vertebro-basilar trunk is seen in the left cerebello-pontine angle.

2. Lesions Involving the Fourth Ventricle

(i)   Non-visualization   — poor scan quality (normal)
                                        — compression by local mass
                                        — occupied by isodense blood
                                        — isodense tumour (unusual)

(ii)   Raised attenuation without deformity — intraventricular blood
                                        (Fig. 11.5)

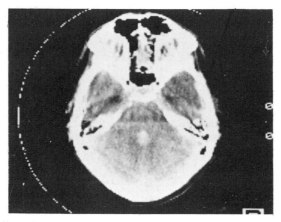

Fig. 11.5   Blood within the fourth ventricle.

(iii) Masses involving the fourth ventricle
    (a) *Greater than brain attenuation*
       Medulloblastoma (predominantly)
       Ependymoma (usually)
       Astrocytoma
       Metastasis
       Choroid plexus papilloma

    (b) *Brain attenuation*
       Ependymoma
       Medulloblastoma
       Metastasis
    (c) *Less than brain attenuation*
       Dermoid
       Metastasis
       Astocytoma (usually)

These lesions are seen to be in the position of the fourth ventricle, but it is frequently impossible to determine whether the lesion arises in or adjacent to the ventricle. The fourth ventricle may sometimes be seen dilated around an intrinsic lesion as a halo of CSF attenuation (Fig. 11.6) but frequently the fourth ventricle itself cannot be identified.

N.B. The normal vermis may be of strikingly high attenuation.

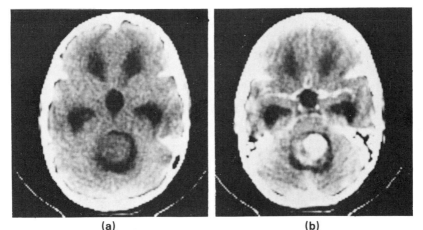

(a)   **(b)**

Fig. 11.6 (a, b) Rounded isodense lesion within the fourth ventricle showing dense enhancement after contrast. Ependymoma.

3. Cerebellar Lesions

(i) High attenuation

Haemorrhage (Fig. 11.7)	– blood attenuation
Haemorrhagic infarct	– mixed high and low attenuation
Medulloblastoma	– midline, well circumscribed
Metastasis	– variable attenuation and enhancement
Astrocytoma	– hemispheric mass

(ii) Brain attenuation

Astrocytoma	– usually accompanied by surrounding oedema.
Infarct	– occasionally isodense
Metastasis	– usually accompanied by surrounding oedema

(iii) Low attenuation

Astocytoma (Fig. 11.8)   – typically low density
Haemangioblastoma (Fig. 11.9) – ring + nodule, may be solid, multiple, very small
Metastasis
Abscess (Fig. 11.10)   – ring enhancement
Infarct (Fig. 11.11)   – with or without mass effect

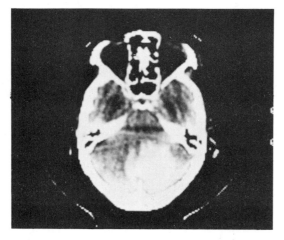

Fig. 11.7 Right cerebellar hemisphere haemorrhage.

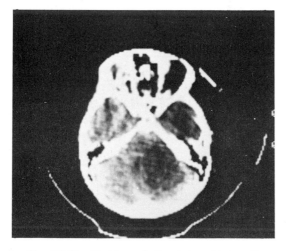

Fig. 11.8 Right cerebellar astrocytoma, displacing the fourth ventricle.

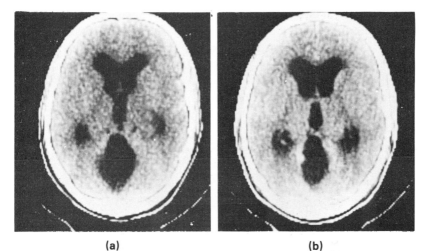

(a) **(b)**

Fig. 11.9 (a) Haemangioblastoma: Unenhanced scan showing low attentuation cyst in the region of the superior vermis.
(b) Small enhancing mural nodule following contrast injection.

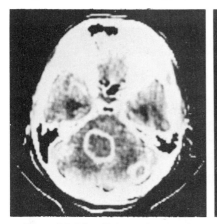
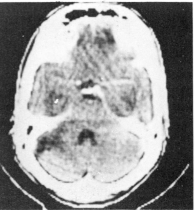

Fig. 11.10 Tuberculous abscesses: ring enhancement following contrast injection.

Fig. 11.11 Left cerebellar hemisphere low attenuation without mass effect. The fourth ventricle is undisplaced. Cerebellar infarct.

A well circumscribed low attenuation lesion is usually a cystic astrocytoma or a haemangioblastoma, but may be a metastasis. Metastasis is the most frequent lesion in adults and may be multiple. Ring enhancement suggests abscess. The posterior fossa is a difficult area and lesions may only be detected on plain scans by subtle displacements of the fourth ventricle and cisterns. Contrast enhancement is probably obligatory if a posterior fossa lesion is suspected. An uncommon cause of a low attenuation cyst particularly in children is the Dandy-Walker syndrome, caused by a membranous obstruction to the outlet of the fourth ventricle. There is associated cerebellar hypoplasia.

4. Lesions of Brainstem

High attenuation
  Haemorrhage (Fig. 11.12)
  Tumour   – unusual
  Angioma   – uncommon
Low attenuation
  Tumour (Fig. 11.13)   – glioma is usually low attenuation
  Infarct   – difficult to demonstrate
Brainstem infarcts are notoriously difficult to demonstrate due to frequent artefact in this region.

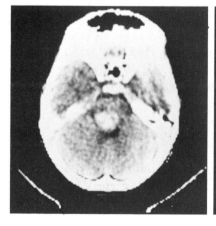   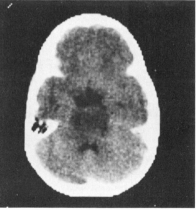

Fig. 11.12 Unenhanced scan showing posterior pontine high attenuation. Spontaneous brainstem haemorrhage.

Fig. 11.13 Low attenuation brainstem swelling. Glioma.

NOTES ON COMMON POSTERIOR FOSSA LESIONS

(a) Acoustic Neuroma

This tumour is characterized by its situation at the internal auditory meatus (which can be visualized on the scan at high window width). It is usually isodense with the adjacent brain and is frequently invisible prior to contrast enhancement, although some deformity of the fourth ventricle is often seen. There may be low attenuation in the compressed but oedematous cerebellum. The tumour almost always enhances with intravenous contrast.

(b) Cerebellar Tumours

Cerebellar tumours are hemispheric or midline (vermian) masses. In adults the commonest tumours are metastases, which may be multiple. Their attenuation is very variable and oedema is usually present. They may be solid or cystic. When solitary it is virtually impossible to differentiate them from primary cerebellar tumours. For practical purposes the patient's age and history are the best guide.

Astrocytoma. Astrocytoma has a variable pattern; it is most often seen as a low attenuation cystic area in the cerebellar hemisphere. It may, however, be of raised or mixed attenuation. These tumours often enhance.

Medulloblastoma. This is a midline lesion which arises in the region of the inferior vermis. It is normally isodense or of slightly raised attenuation, slightly irregular in outline, and enhances. It frequently metastasises through the CSF pathways. It tends to present as a hemisphere mass in adults.

Ependymoma. This is a midline tumour arising in the fourth ventricle, usually isodense but may contain calcification or haemorrhage. It usually shows quite marked enhancement.

Haemangioblastoma. Haemangioblastoma classically appears as a low attenuation cystic lesion which sometimes bears a mural nodule which enhances or presents as an enhancing ring of tumour around a cyst. They may be small, solid and multiple. It is often indistinguishable from a cystic astrocytoma.

(c) Brainstem Tumour

Swelling of the brainstem is indicated by encroachment on, or effacement of, the surrounding CSF spaces, including the fourth ventricle which may be displaced and deformed (Fig. 11.14). Attenuation abnormality is usually slight, most frequently being less than brain attenuation. Enhancement is rarely striking, frequently absent.

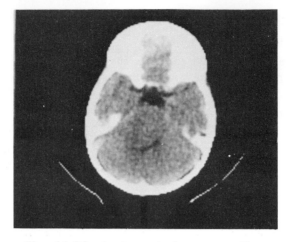

Fig. 11.14   Isodense brainstem swelling. The brainstem is expanded and is displacing the deformed fourth ventricle posteriorly. Glioma.

CHAPTER TWELVE

Bone

Although the spatial resolving power of CT does not yet equal that of conventional radiography, CT may be applied to lesions affecting the skull base and vault. CT simultaneously displays bone structure and detail of the adjacent intra- and extracranial soft tissues. Manipulation of window level and width allows detail of bone or of soft tissue to be viewed preferentially from the same slice. The commonly employed settings for bone are a level of + 100 HU and a window width of + 400 HU.

The observations made when viewing bone detail may for practical purposes be discussed in terms of bone deformity, thickening, thinning and defect. The full radiological picture of any condition frequently includes a mixture of these changes. Some of the commoner lesions are tabulated below:

1. Bone Deformity

Sellar expansion

Pituitary tumour — contains soft tissue
Empty sella — cerebrospinal fluid attenuation
Optic chiasm tumour — excavation in the region of the sulcus chiasmaticus
Aneurysm — usually eccentric erosion of sphenoid bone (Fig. 12.1)
Raised intracranial pressure — dilated third ventricle in sella
Neurofibromatosis — as part of the dysplasia seen in this condition

Enlarged orbit

Neurofibromatosis — due to deficient sphenoid wing (dysplasia), — macrophthalmia or neurofibromatous tissue

Sinus expansion

Neoplastic — soft tissue mass with destruction of bony walls
Mucocele — thin but intact bony margins
Rarely inflammatory polyps — thin but intact bony margins

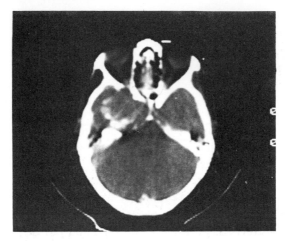

Fig. 12.1   Wide window image showing erosion of the left side of the sphenoid bone and amputation of the left anterior clinoid process by a giant carotid aneurysm. Calcification in its wall present in the middle fossa.

2. Bone thickening

Localized changes

Fibrous dysplasia — CT may show fibrous intradiploic component

(Absence of an associated soft tissue mass helps distinguish from meningioma.)

Meningioma — hyperostosis at site of attachment. CT shows extent of associated mass. Bone may be infiltrated and thickened without intracranial mass.

Epidermoid — CT shows intradiploic expansion, soft tissue attenuation contents, clear-cut margins.

Expanding deposit — metastasis — irregular margins and some-
— myeloma   times soft tissue swelling indicate destructive nature.

Others: Paget's disease (Fig. 12.2)
Simple enostosis
Simple exostosis
Cephalhaematoma — calcified/ossified

Diffuse changes

Secondary to arrested or impaired brain development
Paget's disease
Osteopetrosis
Cerebral Hemiatrophy   — thickened calvarium of smaller volume hemicranium, extensive sinus pneumatization on affected side.

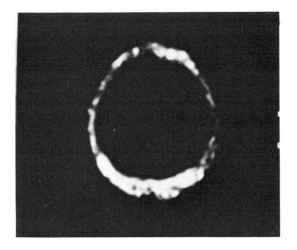

Fig. 12.2 Wide window image of calvarium showing bone expansion with 'lucent' areas. Paget's disease.

3. Bone Thinning

Localized changes:

Arachnoid cyst   — if in contact with vault. (CT shows erosion
Epidermoid   — of bone as well as the intracranial mass).

Chronic subdural haematoma
Tumour (occasionally)

Diffuse changes:

Secondary to Chronic   — may be calcified.
subdural haematoma

4. Bone Defects

(a) *Skull base*

Fracture	– axial display of anatomy is useful
Acoustic neuroma	– erosion of the internal auditory canal (Fig. 12.3)
Fifth nerve neuroma	– petrous apex erosion
Ninth nerve neuroma	– jugular foramen erosion
Glomus jugulare tumour	– jugular foramen erosion (Fig. 12.4)
Nasopharyngeal carcinoma	– may erode sphenoid bone
Chordoma	– erosion of clivus region

(b) *Vault*

Fracture
Metastasis, myeloma
Inflammatory lesions
Radionecrosis
Surgical defects

NB: Sutures and fontanelles are seen as normal defects in appropriate age groups.

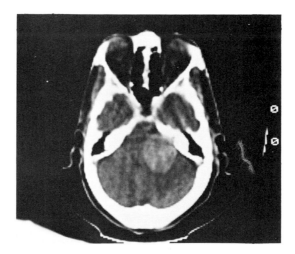

Fig. 12.3 Wide window image showing expanded internal auditory meatus and large acoustic neuroma.

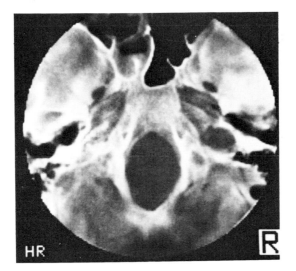

Fig. 12.4 Expansion of the right jugular foramen. (High resolution technique.) Glomus jugulare tumour.

CHAPTER THIRTEEN

The Orbit

Intraorbital Masses – classified according to site

1. Extraconal lesions   – outside the cone formed by the extra-ocular muscles
2. Extra-ocular muscle enlargement
3. Intraconal lesions
4. Optic nerve lesions

INTRAORBITAL MASSES

1. Extraconal Lesions

Encroachment from sinuses	– mucocoele (Fig. 13.1)
	– carcinoma
	– haemangiofibroma
	– polyp (rarely)
Bony encroachment	– fibrous dysplasia
	– meningioma
	– metastasis
Lacrimal gland mass	– granuloma
	– tumour
Tumours	– metastasis, lymphoma
	– epidermoid and dermoid

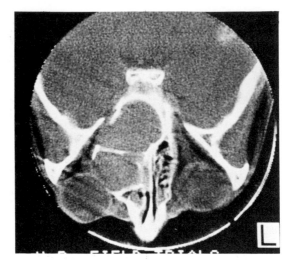

Fig. 13.1 Soft tissue mass in the right ethmoidal sinus expanding into the orbit. Right ethmoid mucocoele.

2. Extra-ocular Muscle Enlargement

Thyroid eye disease (Fig. 13.2)	— frequently bilateral — spectrum of affection, from a solitary muscle to all muscles — muscle bellies particularly swollen
Orbital granuloma	— often with patchy increase in attenuation of orbital fat, or discrete mass
Carotico-cavernous fistula	— may see large veins in orbit

'Myositis'

3. Intraconal Lesions

Cavernous haemangioma (Fig. 13.3)	— well defined mass, commonest lesion
Granuloma (pseudo-tumour)	— discrete mass or ill defined, patchy increase in attenuation of orbital fat. Frequently associated with sinus disease.
Varix/arteriovenous malformation	— irregular shape
'Hypertrophy' of fat	— chronic thyroid eye disease

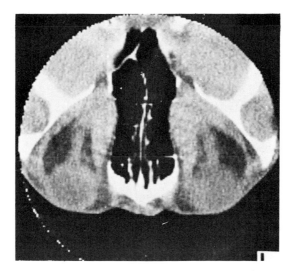

(a)

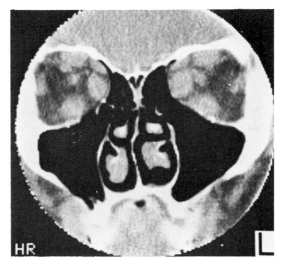

(b)

Fig. 13.2 (a) Bilateral extra-ocular muscle swelling. Thyroid eye disease. Compare to normal scan p. 31.
(b) Coronal scan.

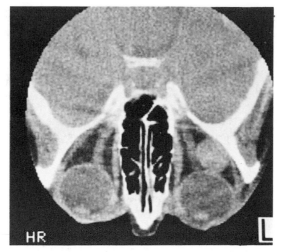

Fig. 13.3   Well-defined spherical mass in left muscle cone. Cavernous haemangioma.

4. Optic Nerve Lesions

Swelling — nerve sheath meningioma (Fig. 13.4)
— glioma (Fig. 13.5)
— papilloedema
— possibly in optic neuritis

Thinning — optic atrophy
— stretched nerves (proptosis)

Cavernous haemangioma is by far the commonest intraconal mass. It is usually very well defined, oval or spherical. It is most commonly situated in the infero-lateral quadrant of the muscle cone, but may show marked mobility from one scan to another. When very large, there may be associated orbital expansion.

Optic nerve sheath meningioma usually causes a diffuse thickening with slight elongation of the nerve which is of somewhat increased attenuation, sometimes calcified. Occasionally, there may be detectable hyperostosis at the orbital apex.

Optic nerve glioma typically causes a fusiform swelling of the nerve which may indent the back of the globe. It may be bilateral and extend to the optic chiasm in the suprasellar region, in which case the optic canal may be shown to be widened. It only exceptionally contains calcification before irradiation.

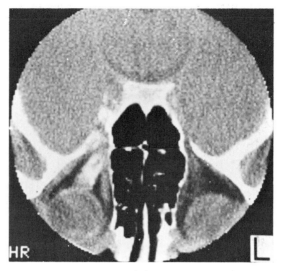

(a)

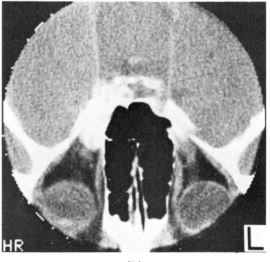

(b)

Fig. 13.4 (a) + (b)   Thickened right optic nerve with calcification. The tumour extends through the optic canal to the parasellar region. Optic nerve sheath meningioma.

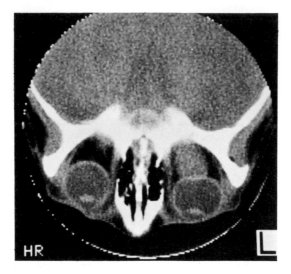

Fig. 13.5 Fusiform optic nerve swelling slightly indenting the back of the left globe. Optic nerve glioma.

CHAPTER FOURTEEN

The Post-operative Scan

One of the most important contributions of CT scanning has been in the management of the post-operative neurosurgical patient, especially in the first few hours or days following operation. A patient who has undergone neurosurgery is in an unstable state and is liable to a variety of complications, whose management calls for early accurate diagnosis. Distinguishing, for example, an accumulating haematoma which may require evacuation from brain swelling or infarction which calls for conservative management is frequently impossible by clinical methods, but since the advent of CT it is possible to reach a prompt and accurate diagnosis in most cases.

1. The early postoperative period

The patient is at greatest risk in the first days immediately after surgery. Deterioration in the patient's level of consciousness or other clinical signs is usually an indication for a CT scan which may show some of the following features:

(a) *Haemorrhage:* this may be a local haemorrhage at the operative site, or a haematoma in the region of the craniotomy. These findings are relative indications for re-exploration, depending on the size of the haematoma and the patient's condition. A significant haematoma usually causes visible mass effect.

(b) *Brain swelling, ischaemia and infarction:* isodense swelling of one or both hemispheres may be seen on the postoperative scan; transient swelling following surgery may be amenable to steroid therapy. Brain swelling may, however, result from ischaemia, and it must be distinguished from an isodense subdural haematoma. The term ischaemia implies a potentially reversible vascular lesion, either due to spasm or transient arterial occlusion. It may be seen on the postoperative CT scan as an area of isodense swelling, or as an area of reduced attenuation. A low attenuation area following surgery, especially in the presence of arterial spasm, does not therefore always signify infarction, and the CT lesion and associated clinical deficit may be reversible, sometimes calling for the use of hypertensive agents. Infarcted tissue may remain isodense for a few days. Such a lesion may enhance with injected contrast medium, but contrast enhancement has a limited role in this situation as it is potentially toxic, and may further harm already damaged tissue.

(c) *Residual tumour:* high attenuation at the site of a resected lesion may be due to haematoma or blood absorbed by surgical foam and may be misinterpreted as a residual tumour.

(d) *Postoperative changes only:* craniotomy, surgical clips at the operation site and either limited local damage due to surgery or a cavity left by a tumour may be seen. Local damage to an evocative area of the brain may be shown and suggest the cause of deterioration; isodense ischaemia should be considered when no obvious cause is apparent.

2. Delayed Complications

The complications mentioned above are not always restricted to the first few post-operative days. Development of hydrocephalus or infection tends to occur a little later.

(a) *Hydrocephalus:* may have been present pre-operatively, and if so would usually have been treated by shunting prior to any major procedure. Communicating hydrocephalus may, however, result from operation, due to the interference in CSF absorption by subarachnoid blood from haemorrhage at operation.

(b) *Infection:* may be seen intracerebrally or extracerebrally. In the former, marked ring enhancement suggests this possibility. Infected extracerebral collections usually show marked marginal enhancement, representing the thickened meninges forming a 'capsule'.

3. Tumour Recurrence and Radiotherapy

When a lesion has been completely removed at surgery, the scan usually shows an area of low attenuation localized to that site, representing damaged brain or surgical cavity. Local atrophy with dilatation of the adjacent part of the ventricular system develops subsequently.

Recurrence of a previously excised lesion frequently has the attenuation and enhancement characteristics of the original lesion. Contrast injection should be performed when looking for a recurrence, as the contribution to the scan appearance by operative changes makes assessment very difficult.

Positive detection of a recurrence is frequently difficult in patients who have been subjected to radiotherapy, since this treatment may give rise to features that are indistinguishable by CT from recurrent tumour. However, irradiation typically gives rise to local atrophy at the site of radiation, sometimes accompanied by more diffuse atrophy in the rest of the brain. Irradiation may also induce the formation of granulomata which may have mass effect and show enhancement after contrast, simulating tumour recurrence.

CHAPTER FIFTEEN

Clinical Correlation

This section comprises notes on the commoner neurological terms which may be encountered in CT work. A brief definition is given followed by an indication of the common causative pathologies and their possible sites. The list is not exhaustive and is intended as a practical aid to be used in conjunction with CT, rather than as a comprehensive list of clinical diagnoses: conditions which are not detected by CT scan are therefore largely excluded.

Abducens Nerve Palsy – The sixth cranial nerve passes from the pons to the orbit traversing the cavernous sinus and passing through the superior orbital fissure. A palsy may be caused by a lesion compressing the nerve anywhere along its course, or by raised intracranial pressure.

Acalculia – a defect in the use of numerals.

Agnosia– is a failure of recognition of a stimulus, visual, tactile or auditory in the presence of sufficient vision, feeling or hearing. These defects usually occur in parietal or temporal lobe disease.

Agraphia – a defect in the production of written language.

Akinesia – slowness of movement typical of Parkinson's disease.

Alexia – a defect in the comprehension of written language.

Amaurosis fugax – sudden transient loss of vision lasting less than 24 hours (*see* Vision, disorders of).

Amnesia – severe memory loss. May occur in presenile and senile dementias, e.g. Alzheimer's, cerebral atherosclerosis or in severe head injury. It may also occur in tumours in the region of the IIIrd ventricle.

Anosmia – loss of sense of smell. May be caused by a lesion of the floor of anterior fossa, typically a meningioma.

Aphasia – a defect of language. The characteristics may suggest the localization as in Broca's which is localized to the dominant posterior inferior frontal lobe, and in Wernicke's localized to the posterior one third of the dominant superior temporal gyrus.

Apraxia – inability to carry out a purposeful movement in the absence of difficulty in comprehension, motor or sensory defect, or ataxia. It usually indicates parietal lobe or association fibre disease.

Astereognosis – a specific form of tactile agnosia usually due to a lesion posterior to the post central gyrus.

Ataxia – a disorder of voluntary movement, not due to weakness, causing the break up of normal smooth movement, which may occur in cerebellar disease.

Athetosis – slow writhing movements due to disease of the basal ganglia, often in the putamen.

Babinski sign – extensor plantar reflex; a sign of damage to the contralateral upper motor neurone pathway.

Bulbar palsy – paralysis of muscles of throat and tongue, e.g. by a brainstem tumour.

Cerebellar disorder – the commoner signs that are associated with a lesion of the cerebellum or its connections are: ataxia, intention tremor, dysarthria and nystagmus.

Cheyne-Stokes respiration – a characteristic waxing and waning type of respiration which may occur in large or bilateral supratentorial lesions and in high brainstem lesions.

Chorea – rapid interrupted almost purposeful movements due to disease of the basal ganglia for instance in Huntington's chorea.

Clonus – is a part of the same state of hyperreflexia as spasticity and indicates an upper motor neurone lesion.

Cogwheel rigidity – a change in tone typical of Parkinson's disease.

Coma – some of the numerous causes include the following which may be detected by CT:

1. haemorrhage – intracerebral, cerebellar, subarachnoid, subdural, extradural
2. cerebral or brainstem infarct
3. cerebral or brainstem tumour
4. abscess, encephalitis, meningitis.

Deafness – CT may show a lesion of the middle ear (inflammatory disease, cholesteatoma), the cerebello-pontine angle (e.g. acoustic neuroma) or of the brainstem (tumour, infarct).

Delirium – a disordered mental state with confusion and restless excitement. It is most commonly due to toxic or metabolic causes. It may occur in head injury and encephalitis and infrequently with a mass lesion.

Dementia – deterioration of memory and intellect.

The causes include:

1. cerebral degeneration, e.g. Alzheimer's

2. cerebrovascular disease – multi-infarct
3. tumour – with or without raised intracranial pressure.

Diabetes insipidus – passage of large volumes of urine usually due to interference with anti-diuretic hormone (ADH) secretion. Tumours of the hypothalamic region and basal meningitis which are occasional causes may be seen on the scan.

Dysarthria – a disorder of articulation of speech. May be due to a paresis of the muscles of the throat or tongue of lower motor neurone (bulbar palsy) or upper motor neurone (pseudobulbar palsy) type. It may also be caused by a cerebellar lesion (q.v.) or a lesion of the basal ganglia (e.g. Parkinson's disease).

Dysphasia – (*see* aphasia)

Dystonia – slow sustained twisting movement involving the face, trunk or limbs and is due to disease of the basal ganglia.

Epilepsy – this may be idiopathic or symptomatic of an underlying disorder which may be seen on CT. The main types of epilepsy are:

1. 'Grand mal' or generalized epilepsy, with loss of consciousness
2. 'Petit mal' or momentary absence attacks
3. Focal epilepsy – attacks arising in a localized part of the brain but may either remain localized or spread to give a generalized fit.

A Jacksonian seizure is a form of focal epilepsy starting usually in thumb and index finger or angle of the mouth or the great toe which then spreads. 'Grand mal' and more frequently focal epilepsy may be symptomatic of an underlying cerebral lesion depending on the age of the patient. Possible scan abnormalities include:

    congenital disorders – birth injury and infarction
    trauma
    tumour
    infection – abscess, encephalitis, toxoplasmosis, cysticercosis
    infarction and vascular disease
    degenerative disease.

Exophthalmos – protrusion of one or both eyes. Possible causes include:

    dysthyroid eye disease
    granuloma/pseudotumour
    neurofibromatosis
    optic nerve glioma
    optic sheath meningioma
    cavernous haemangioma
    metastasis
    cavernous sinus lesions (e.g. thrombosis).

Facial palsy – of the upper motor neurone type is clinically distinguishable from that caused by a lower motor neurone lesion. The former may occur with any supranuclear lesion, the latter with a nuclear or peripheral lesion. Commonest causes of a lower motor neurone lesion which may be seen on CT are:

    pontine tumour or infarct

    cerebellopontine angle lesion (e.g. acoustic neuroma)

    basilar aneurysm.

Focal epilepsy – (*see* epilepsy)

Frontal lobe syndromes – lesions in the frontal lobe may cause personality change, lack of concentration and initiative and loss of social behaviour. Anosmia may be caused by inferior frontal lesions. Other occasional findings are: grasp and sucking reflexes, a gaze palsy, urinary difficulties or pyramidal weakness.

Gaze palsy – loss of conjugate eye movements in any one direction due to a lesion of the supranuclear fibres at any point in their course.

Gerstmann's syndrome – a combination of right-left disorientation, acalculia, finger agnosia and agraphia, caused by a lesion in the region of the dominant angular gyrus.

Grand mal epilepsy – (*see* epilepsy)

Hallucinations – auditory hallucinations occur in temporal lobe epilepsy, or in association with a temporal lobe lesion (e.g. tumour) and rarely in pontine lesions. Visual hallucinations can be produced by lesions in the occipital lobe or posterior temporal lobe. Hallucinations of smell occur in temporal lobe epilepsy with or without an underlying structural lesion.

Headache – is a frequent non-specific accompaniment of intracranial disorder. It is, however, not an indication in itself for CT scanning.

Hemianopia – (*see* visual field defects)

Hemiballismus – violent 'flinging' movements, due to a lesion in the subthalamic region.

Hemiplegia – weakness of one half of the body due to a lesion of the corticospinal tract often in the internal capsule. Any lesion may be responsible but vascular disease (i.e. infarction) is the most frequent.

Horner's Syndrome – (*see* pupillary abnormalities) is due to paralysis of the sympathetic nerve supply causing a relatively smaller pupil, ptosis of the lid, apparent enophthalmos with absence of sweating.

Hyperventilation – deep, rapid respiration which may be due to a lesion in the lower midbrain or upper pons or may be due to transtentorial herniation.

Hypoglossal palsy – (XII cranial nerve) causes paralysis of the tongue musculature. It may be part of an upper motor neurone lesion, or a lower motor neurone lesion at medullary level or peripherally (e.g. jugular foramen).

Inappropriate ADH secretion – retention of water due to secretion of excessive antidiuretic hormone. Neurological causes include a cerebral tumour, abscess and infarct, as well as subarachnoid haemorrhage and trauma.

Intention tremor – a form of tremor brought on and intensified by movement, often seen in cerebellar disease.

Internuclear ophthalmoplegia – causes dissociation of conjugate lateral gaze so that there is slowing or failure of the adducting eye with nystagmus usually seen in the abducting eye. It indicates involvement of the medial longitudinal fasciculus.

Jacksonian epilepsy – (*see* epilepsy).

Korsakow's psychosis – severe defect of memory for recent events in association with confabulation.

L'Hermitte's sign – tingling sensation down the back on flexing the neck, implies cervical or foramen magnum lesion.

Mental retardation – subnormal intelligence, from birth or apparent in early life. The cause may sometimes be genetic or hereditary and occasionally the scan will show an abnormality (e.g. in tuberose sclerosis). Acquired causes include: intrauterine infection (calcification may be seen intracranially in toxoplasmosis, cytomegalic inclusion disease), or a traumatic event at birth (scan may show atrophy or porencephaly).

Migraine – a common condition which may rarely be a symptom of underlying angioma or aneurysm.

Monoplegia – weakness of one limb (*see* movement, disorders of).

Movement disorders – movement may be impaired in several ways: (a) Paralysis or paresis may be due to an upper motor neurone lesion affecting any part of the motor pathway from the cortex to the nucleus of a peripheral nerve, or to a lower motor neurone lesion affecting the cranial or peripheral nerves at any point from the brainstem or spinal cord to the muscles they supply. A lesion of the cortex may cause monoparesis. In the corona radiata or internal capsule, hemiparesis is more likely due to the concentration of fibres. (In the latter, sensory and visual symptoms are also often present.) In the brainstem, cranial nerves may be affected as they leave the brainstem resulting in a lower motor neurone lesion.

Movements may also be impaired by:
(b) a basal ganglia disorder
(c) a cerebellar disorder

(d) a sensory deficit

(e) apraxia.

Myoclonus – this is a short shock-like contraction of muscles, often seen in patients with epilepsy. It is occasionally associated with rare dementing disorders, or occasionally with encephalitis.

Nystagmus – is a disorder of eye movements showing rhythmic involuntary oscillations. Particular types of nystagmus can be distinguished and may be of localizing value.

Occipital lobe symptoms – a lesion of one occipital lobe will cause a contralateral homonymous field defect if it affects visual cortex or optic radiation. Other symptoms which may result include visual agnosia and visual hallucinations.

Optic atrophy – or optic disc pallor (on ophthalmoscopy) is due to loss of nerve fibres at the optic disc.

Causes include:

Optic neuritis (usually due to multiple sclerosis)

optic nerve tumour

occlusive vascular disease

chronic papilloedema

Orbital lesions – (*see* exophthalmos)

Papilloedema – swelling of the optic disc seen on ophthalmoscopy. It can be due to raised intracranial pressure from any cause:

tumour

hydrocephalus

abscess

subarachnoid haemorrhage

venous sinus thrombosis

infection – encephalitis, meningitis

benign intracranial hypertension

hypertensive encephalopathy.

Paraplegia – bilateral leg weakness usually due to bilateral upper motor neurone lesions, usually in the spinal cord, but occasionally caused by a parasagittal intracranial lesion, most commonly meningioma.

Parietal lobe symptoms – include sensory disturbance, occasionally with neglect of the affected side. Pain and temperature sensitivity are usually preserved. A lesion of the dominant parietal lobe may cause aphasia or any of the features of Gerstmann's syndrome (q.v.). A lesion of the non-dominant parietal lobe may cause constructional or dressing apraxia.

Parkinsonism – Parkinson's disease is a degenerative disorder of the basal ganglia whose predominant symptoms are:

akinesia
cogwheel rigidity of the limbs
resting tremor.
A scan may rarely show a lesion of the basal ganglia in Parkinson's disease. Symptoms like those seen in Parkinson's disease may occur in other diseases of the basal ganglia, pseudobulbar palsy, tumour, Wilson's disease or juvenile Huntington's chorea, all of which may produce scan abnormalities. A similar but distinct clinical picture may also be seen in low pressure hydrocephalus.

Precocious puberty – may be caused by a pinealoma or a lesion originating in the hypothalamus.

Pseudobulbar palsy – (*see* dysarthria) due to bilateral upper motor neurone lesions.

Pupillary abnormalities – may be caused by an orbital lesion, optic nerve lesion, a lesion affecting the 3rd nerve (*see* strabismus) or a lesion in the midbrain (pinealoma, multiple sclerosis). Horner's syndrome may be caused by a hypothalamic or a brainstem lesion.

Sensory symptoms – may be caused by intracranial lesions situated anywhere between the brainstem and the cortex. In the pons or medulla a lesion may cause a 'crossed' clinical syndrome of loss of pain and temperature on one side of the face and the opposite side of the body. A lesion in the thalamus causes decreased or loss of sensation in the opposite half of the body; occasionally a thalamic syndrome may result. A lesion in the posterior limb of the internal capsule will cause a hemisensory loss. In the parietal lobe, a lesion may cause discriminatory sensory functions to be lost: localization of touch, position – sense or ability to distinguish two simultaneous bilateral stimuli (inattention).

Spasm, hemifacial – a recurrent spasm of one side of the face – occasional cases are said to be caused by a tortuous or ectatic vessel compressing the facial nerve in the posterior fossa.

Spasticity – an increase in muscle tone with brisk tendon reflexes due to an upper motor neurone lesion.

Strabismus (squint) – is the failure of normal co-ordination of the ocular axes. A paralytic strabismus must be distinguished from a concomitant strabismus. The following lesions may give rise to a paralytic strabismus:
Orbital lesion – (*see* exophthalmos)
Orbital apex lesion:
   meningioma
   Paget's disease
Parasellar lesions:

pituitary adenoma
aneurysm
craniopharyngioma
nasopharyngeal carcinoma
fracture of skull base
uncal herniation (tentorial coning)
Brainstem:
infarction
tumour (pinealoma, glioma).

Stroke – sudden onset of cerebral dysfunction, usually due to an infarct or haemorrhage.

Syncope – transient loss of consciousness due to cerebral hypoxia. It is not usually related to intracranial disease.

Syndromes:

Anton's – visual deficit with denial of this by the patient, caused by occipital lesions extending to association areas.

Foster-Kennedy – optic atrophy in one eye with papilloedema in the other, often due to meningioma in parasellar region.

Gerstmann's – (q.v.)

Horner's – (q.v.)

Shy-Drager – degenerative disorder with extrapyramidal symptoms and failure of autonomic functions.

Steel-Richardson-Olszewski – (progressive supranuclear palsy). A degenerative disorder with supranuclear ophthalmoplegia, pseudo-bulbar palsy and axial dystonia.

Thalamic – (q.v.)

Tolosa-Hunt – painful ophthalmoplegia, orbital pain, decreased eye movement, 5th nerve sensory loss – cavernous sinus lesion.

Temporal lobe symptoms – a frequent manifestation of a lesion of the temporal lobe is epilepsy (q.v.) sometimes with uncinate fits with disturbance of taste and smell. Other symptoms are: auditory hallucinations, an upper homonymous quadrantinopia and occasionally aggressive behaviour. A lesion of the dominant temporal lobe may cause aphasia and bilateral lesions can cause memory disturbance, disordered sexual function and apathy.

Thalamic syndrome – severe often burning pain in one half of the body due to a thalamic lesion.

Transient ischaemic attack – sudden transient cerebral dysfunction lasting 24 hours. Sometimes a sign of carotid embolic disease. Scan usually normal.

Trigeminal neuralgia – characteristic shooting pain in the face. Rarely caused by a posterior fossa tumour (e.g. acoustic neuroma). Also a rare symptom of multiple sclerosis.

Vertigo – feeling of loss of balance with sensation of rotation usually due to middle ear disease but a brainstem or cerebellar lesion may cause this symptom.

Visual disorders – the pattern of visual field loss (*see* visual field defect) or evolution of the disorder may suggest the cause. Gradual monocular visual loss suggests a compressive lesion of the optic nerve. Sudden bilateral blindness may be due to bilateral occipital lobe infarction. The causative lesion may often be apparent on CT scan:

orbit – *see* exophthalmos
orbital apex
   meningioma
   bone disease
sellar region
   pituitary adenoma (usually bitemporal hemianopia)
   craniopharyngioma (usually bitemporal hemianopia)
   aneurysm
   granulomatous meningitis
retrochiasmatic
   tumour
   infarct
   abscess

Visual field defects – may be homonymous where the same half of the visual field of both eyes (e.g. both right halves) is affected indicating retrochiasmatic involvement or heteronymous where the opposite halves of the visual field of both eyes are affected (e.g. both nasal halves) indicating a lesion in the region of the chiasm. The field loss additionally may be hemianopic involving one half, quadrantinopic involving one quarter or scotomatous involving an area enclosed within the visual field.

Index